MITOCHONDRIAL DYSFUNCTION

A Functional Medicine Approach to Diagnosis and Treatment

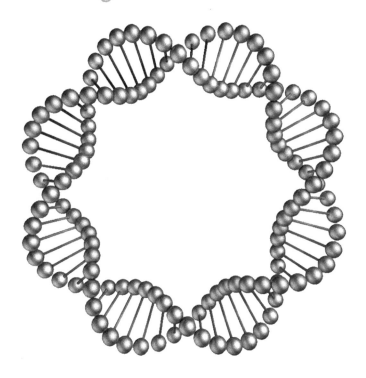

Get Rid of Fat, Fatigue, and Brain Fog

MICHAEL T. CHANG, MD

First edition: August 2019

Cover Design by 100Covers.com
Interior Design by FormattedBooks.com

ISBN 978-1-7333973-1-5

Printed in the United States of America

www.healedandwhole.com
drchang@healedandwhole.com

PRAISE FOR
MITOCHONDRIAL DYSFUNCTION: A FUNCTIONAL MEDICINE APPROACH TO DIAGNOSIS AND TREATMENT

"In his new book *Mitochondrial Dysfunction: A Functional Medicine Approach to Diagnosis and Treatment* Dr. Michael Chang outlines the pressing health concerns that arise from dysfunction of our energy-producing systems. With obesity, depression and metabolic disorders like diabetes so dramatically on the rise a new paradigm for understanding how to treat these conditions is imperative and Dr. Chang presents solutions to these real-world problems. Based on relatively new science and recent discoveries in laboratory testing using functional medicine he shows us clearly how these problems develop and what can be done to assess and correct mitochondrial problems. I found the book a fascinating journey into an area we all would do well to learn more about.

—Dan Kalish, founder of Kalish Institute, IFM faculty

"It was a privilege to interview Dr. Chang for my podcast The Energy Blueprint. I highly recommend picking up a copy of his book *"Mitochondrial Dysfunction: A Functional Medicine Approach to Diagnosis and Treatment."* I had an advance copy and found it excellent. **Highly recommended.**"

—Ari Whitten, The Energy Blueprint

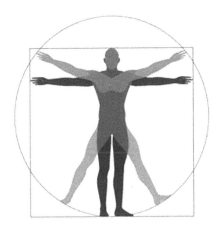

THANK YOU FOR PURCHASING THIS BOOK.
I HOPE YOU ENJOY IT.

Get a FREE ebook "Seven Days to Better Health"
and a summary of this book chapter by chapter
that you can easily review.

You will also get updates on new releases,
free health tips, and my newsletter.

To sign up, please visit www.healedandwhole.com.

CONTENTS

INTRODUCTION

When I began my medical career as a pathologist in the late 1980s, my understanding of mitochondria was limited to what I had learned in college. It is an organelle within every cell and it produces energy for the cell to use for all its activities. I had seen electron microscopy pictures and assumed they were always working in the cell. By 2012, when I was certified as a functional medicine practitioner, this picture hadn't changed.

It wasn't until I did a mentorship with Dr. Dan Kalish that my understanding of the importance of the mitochondria started to change. Since functional medicine is about finding the root cause of a patient's symptoms, I began to understand that it is often the root cause at the cellular level for most age-related chronic diseases. It can underlie the top five symptoms that most functional medicine practitioners see in their practice: fatigue, overweight and can't lose weight, stressed and depressed, gut problems, and hormone imbalance.

The Kalish method emphasizes the importance of functional lab testing. Test results determine the treatment plan, which means there is no guesswork. A lab test called the organic acids test can show mitochondrial dysfunction or a hypometabolic state. What this means is that the mitochondria in the cells are not metabolizing food into cellular energy called adenosine triphosphate (ATP), the "currency" that fuels all cellular functions (all cells use ATP for energy).

There are now many effective treatments using diet, supplements, and lifestyle to reboot the lagging mitochondria or to shut them down and make new ones. When cellular energy is renewed or revitalized, the top five symptoms will improve and eventually be eliminated. Not only will you feel better but you can prevent or delay the onset of many chronic degenerative diseases from occurring in the first place. This is where functional medicine can shine: using predictive lab markers early enough to prevent or delay the onset of chronic disease and extend the productive lifespan of the patient.

When I refer to patients who have seen improvements in their lives, I include myself, as I healed myself using the same therapies that you're about to learn from this book. More people need to know that there are solutions to your set of symptoms that conventional medicine is ill-equipped to deal with. For example, doctors may prescribe pills for relief from symptoms while leave root causes unaddressed.

By the time you have finished reading this book, you will have hope again. You can reach your goals and dreams in life again that the medical system has robbed you of. You can have the energy to dance at your son's or daughter's wedding. Or play with your grandkids and go on that dream vacation. It's all possible because we can recharge that rundown cellular battery called the mitochondria.

MY HEALTH JOURNEY

In the fall of 2016 I began to feel pain and weakness in the right leg particularly when I climbed stairs. I had to hang onto the railing and pull myself up. It led to pain and difficulty walking for any length of time, especially in cold weather. By November, during a trip to Ireland, my legs went into spasms of stiffness and pain. I had to use anti-inflammatories many times a day, something I don't like to do. Luckily it was only episodic and I was able to continue my routine of working out at a gym three times a week. However, I wasn't able to use the treadmill without pain. I thought I was just over-exercising, so I backed off—but there was no improvement. At that time, I could barely bend over to pick something up, and tying my shoes was a major chore. I avoided stairs if at all possible.

By summer of 2017, I began to have some back pain in the mornings. Then it dawned on me that the two symptoms were related. An MRI scan showed severe degeneration of lumbar spine with thinning of the discs. The logical conclusion was the leg pain was from compression of the sciatic nerve. The symptoms, however, did not fit, as I never had pain or tingling at rest or loss of vibration even in the toes. A few sessions of physical therapy didn't help much.

That fall I did a stool test and discovered I have sensitivity to gluten. I embarked on a strict gluten-free ketogenic diet and lost ten pounds effortlessly. However, it did not seem to make a difference in leg pain. As a certified gluten specialist, I knew gluten sensitivity can cause muscle and nerve pain. I tried to eliminate all forms of grain in my diet and it didn't seem to make a difference either.

By late December the leg stiffness and pain worsened. It now interfered with my daily activities at home: I live on a hill with two sets of stairs and a steep driveway. The pain also shifted to the left knee, which was very hard to bend. Doing simple chores like washing dishes left my legs stiff and sore and I had to sit to recover.

Fortunately, that winter was quite mild and dry, but the pain persisted while walking. I then met an ear acupuncturist from China who diagnosed me with colon and gallbladder stagnation, which was causing the thigh pain. She placed several seeds in the right ear so that I could press on them to increase blood and qi (energy) flow to the blocked areas. The pain dissipated somewhat through the warm summer, though any hope of a continued lack of pain was dashed when the weather turned cold again, whereupon the pain got worse to an extent where there were times when it felt like I was walking on a raw nerve or a tightly wound muscle. The pain became so bad that I wasn't able to put much pressure on the right leg, which affected my gait and posture. The acupuncturist asked me to stop eating all meat and eggs and even seafood. So now, between a strict gluten-free diet and no meat or animal products, I had a very hard time finding anything to eat besides vegetables. My weight dropped to a record low and I started looking gaunt with muscle atrophy in the leg from not exercising. The fatigue got worse with even short exertions like carrying groceries.

I then decided to do the organic acids test on myself. I was shocked to discover that I had what I'd seen in so many of my patients: low markers of food metabolism and energy production indicative of mitochondrial dysfunction or hypometabolic (underperforming) state. The test also showed the cause: low glutathione, the main antioxidant in the body, and a marker for oxidative stress. This indicated that there were too many free radicals produced in the mitochondria and not enough antioxidants to neutralize them, thereby causing damage to the mitochondria.

That summer I was introduced to hydrogen water after getting acupuncture. As the smallest molecule, hydrogen can easily diffuse through the cell membranes into the mitochondria and quench free radicals which can damage the mitochondria's energy production as well as its DNA and impair other cell functions. Best of all, H_2 is completely safe since it's natural to our body and produced in large amounts by bacteria in our colon. You can find more details about this form of treatment in Chapter Five.

Despite the supplements, hydrogen water, and lifestyle changes, my fatigue and leg pain worsened by fall. My workout routine had to be curtailed by half and all machine weights reduced. I could not do a workout followed by grocery shopping; it had to be one or the other. When I carried the groceries up the stairs to the house, I had to immediately drink and inhale hydrogen, which allowed a quick recovery within minutes. I also got an electric massager for the spasm in the legs and feet. Sitting stopped the pain but it became increasingly difficult to get back up and start walking again without being hunched over.

By November my legs were getting so stiff I discovered I could not sit down on the floor without falling down. Mornings were often bad despite exercising and stretching for a half hour. My legs would improve somewhat by afternoon, thereby enabling me to take a short walk or go to the gym. However, walking on a treadmill was only possible for five minutes—and only when I supported the arms.

In colder weather, the only thing that consistently helped was the sauna. I have a portable infrared sauna at home that I used several times a week. I also had to use the gym sauna before working out to get loosened up. I saw a chiropractor at that time who noted the stiffness in the legs and suggested some mild stretches. Although his treatment didn't help me, his suggestion that it could be muscle-related was a revelation. The aching ankles and calluses on the inside of both feet suggested misalignment of the muscles too. Still, I had a poor understanding of the role of muscles in joint pain because we were never taught this in medical school.

I began checking the Internet for tight psoas muscles—the hip flexors—from prolonged sitting and to see what stretches I could do to relieve the pain. I was shocked to discover that I couldn't do a squat without arm support. I've always had very strong legs and never needed to hold on to anything when doing a squat. Despite all these attempts, I still lacked a systematic approach to stretching.

As the Christmas holidays approached, the situation got worse. I repeated the ear acupuncture but this time there was no change. A colon cleanse had no effect. A five-day fast without meat or animal products did nothing for the leg pain. I even tried a whole-body energy machine, which made the leg muscles tingle but nothing more. Craniosacral therapy had no effect. Red and near-infrared LED therapy felt good because of the heat but I wasn't sure of any specific outcome. The only thing that made me feel better was the far-infrared portable sauna but it was temporary. I was beginning to lose hope and it seemed like my prayers for healing went unanswered.

My usual lifestyle habits and old routines started to change. I avoided going out when possible because getting in and out of the car and walking even short distances left me exhausted. Many days I had to use a cane to give me strength and balance in the legs. Things got so bad that I ended up getting a disability placard so that I wouldn't have to walk far.

Even though I didn't know the exact cause of my problem, I knew the muscle pain and spasm were from damage to my muscle mitochondria and that the decreased production of energy was causing fatigue and weakness. I also understood that the muscle pain that came about because of an increased formation of lactic acid due to an anaerobic (no oxygen) metabolism as opposed to an aerobic metabolism in the mitochondria. But what was the root cause?

I continued doing the basic mitochondria therapy listed in this book. By New Year's Day of 2019, I felt there was a turnaround in my condition. It seemed like a burden lifted on a physical and spiritual level.

During a stay in warm weather in the Philippines, I came across a podcast by Dave Asprey who was interviewing a man who taught the Egoscue method of stretching to relieve pain (the Egoscue method is a postural therapy for misalignment in the body as it loses its designed posture). It made immediate sense to me and I just knew in my heart that this was the right solution to my problem. I began doing those stretches, which seemed to decrease the stiffness in the hips and legs. I also had several sessions of Thai massage that were very helpful to loosen me up and made me realize how sore the calf muscles were. In the warm weather, I could feel my joints loosening up, which in turn made stretching easier. Swimming was also beneficial because of the buoyancy, which meant the legs wouldn't have to bear weight.

Upon my return, I searched out a local practitioner and found Upright Health. I tried some of the stretches on their website and I felt it was helping. Intrigued by their method, I signed up for four sessions of one-on-one training. Although it proved to be quite a challenge to do these exercises, they soon paid off because they were addressing the root cause: a myofascial pain in the hip muscles from sitting too long in front of the computer, a very common problem today for many people. What happens is that some muscles would be stretched too tight while others would be too weak, both of which created an asymmetry that would pull the ankles and feet out of proper alignment. Even my gait had changed because the legs were spread apart from weak adductors. The biggest lesson this exercise taught me was that stretching as much as I could instead of avoiding pain was a way to recondition the muscles and joints. If I had avoided these exercises I would have only made things worse.

After the sessions, I went on a little excursion to test out my walking ability. Everything went really well, and apart from sore ankles and feet I had no hip pain despite walking six to seven hours a day. So I had finally come across a therapy that would treat the root cause and relieve the pressure on the muscles and soft tissues, and allow the mitochondria to recover by making energy aerobically. What's more, the fatigue finally started to diminish once the muscles were reconditioned.

Today, by following the therapies discussed in this book, I'm well on my way to total recovery in my legs. I still do stretch exercises several times a day. In fact, you can do stretching while sitting at your desk or even while driving. As for me, I'm now able to return to the gym and go through my routines like before. I still sit for long stretches to write this book, but now there is frequent movement and breaks and I often stand or do steps in place even while working on the computer.

Since then, I've done a genetic test that shows a variant in two energy genes: SLG25A12 for impaired mitochondrial function and PGC-1alpha for biogenesis (see chapter one for details). This probably contributed to the mitochondrial dysfunction seen in the lab test as well as my fatigue on exertion.

The journey has been long and hard but I realize that God wanted me to learn how to relate better to my patients and their health journeys. The road back to health is never straightforward and has many twists and turns. No matter what the ailment or illness is, if you don't address the root cause, you will not recover.

I firmly believe that with functional medicine you can recover from whatever condition or symptoms you may be suffering from. So don't wait any longer to get rid of your low energy, fatigue, brain fog, and, as a bonus, lose those extra pounds. Go through the book and understand the importance of the mitochondria and how you can improve their function through proper nutrition, supplementation, and lifestyle changes. The main thing is to take action and stay persistent until you achieve results, and you can do so while making sure that any new therapies you may add are doable and affordable.

Remember, it's the base hits that win the ball game, but you've got to start hitting the ball. As with anything, it takes patience and persistence to achieve your goals. Focus on those goals while the going is hard. Find a functional medicine practitioner familiar with mitochondrial dysfunction to guide you through proper testing. You now have a road map. The rest depends on you to put all this information into action. Let's get started on your journey back to vibrant health and energy!

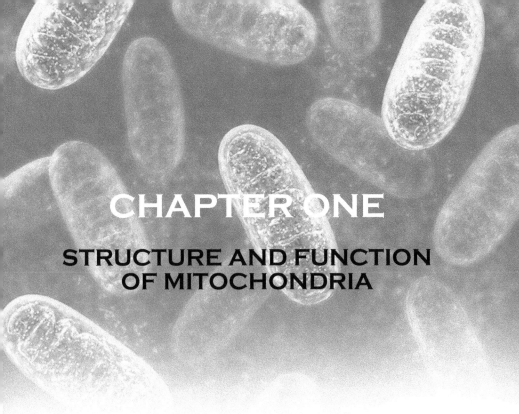

CHAPTER ONE

STRUCTURE AND FUNCTION OF MITOCHONDRIA

Before we can get to diagnosing and treating mitochondrial dysfunction, we need to discuss their structure and normal function. Although the biochemistry of energy production is quite complicated, we will only look at the broad strokes to get a general understanding. We will then look at the various theories of the role mitochondria play in cancer and aging. Finally, we will discuss how mitochondria control autophagy (controlled cell death) and their role in cell regeneration.

CELLULAR STRUCTURE

Mitochondria are the energy factory in every cell that runs all cellular activities. It's like an electric generating plant that runs the appliances in your house. When the generating plant doesn't produce enough electricity, there's a brownout. Similarly, our cells take food, water, and oxygen and convert them to usable energy in the form of adenosine triphosphate (ATP). The mitochondria are the place where this conversion happens.

Mitochondria are cylindrical structures located in the cytoplasm of the cell.

MITOCHONDRIA

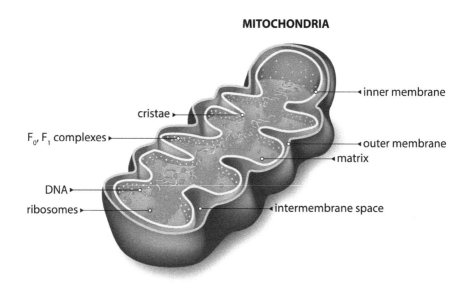

Cross-section structure of mitochondria.

They're able to take many different shapes and are quite flexible. They can divide into two or fuse together. They move around constantly in the cell to where they are needed. Their numbers can range from several hundred to several thousand depending on the activity of the tissue. The heart muscle, skeletal muscle, and brain contain the most number due to the requirement needed for energy. The egg cell of the ovary has one hundred thousand to provide energy to the rapidly dividing embryo after fertilization. Altogether there are about ten million billion mitochondria that make up 10% of the body weight and 50% of the mass of a cell!

Each mitochondrion has a double cell layer. The inner layer is folded to increase the surface area since the energy-making process occurs there. The mitochondrial DNA comes from the mother and is located in the space within the inner membrane. Instead of one copy of DNA in the cell nucleus with forty-six chromosomes, there are several copies of the mitochondrial DNA (mtDNA) that is circular instead of a double helix. It has only thirty-seven genes, which code for the energy assembly line called the electron transport chain (ETC). Furthermore, mtDNA is only inherited from the mother. We can use it to trace a maternal lineage for many generations. When the mitochondria are senescent and dysfunctional, the inner membranes appear thin and ragged under an electron microscope.

MITOCHONDRIAL FUNCTION

Energy Production

The exact mechanism of how energy in the form of ATP is made from food and oxygen is highly complex. Suffice to say the most important function of the mitochondria is aerobic respiration where food is converted to energy requiring oxygen. Digested food is metabolized into energy in three stages.

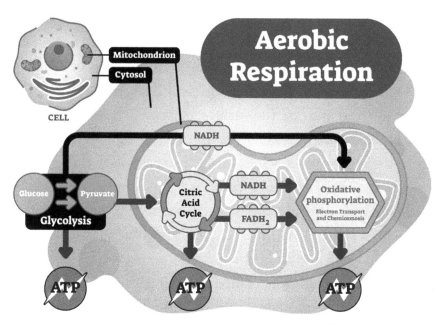

Diagram of aerobic respiration in a cell

Stage I is the breakdown of fats, carbohydrates, and proteins into acetyl CoA and occurs outside the mitochondria. B vitamins, lipoic acid, and carnitine are required in this process. Stage II occurs in the mitochondria where acetyl CoA then enters a series of chemical reactions called the Krebs or citric acid cycle that produce NADH and FADH2, two intermediate energy compounds that donate electrons.

Stage III, called electron transport chain (ETC), takes free electrons of NADH and FADH2 and moves them down a chain of molecules on the inner membrane and combines them with oxygen. This reaction results in the production of water, carbon dioxide, and ATP. This process called oxidative phosphorylation is the reason our bodies stay alive. Each mitochondrion has about ten thousand ETCs and the number can change according to need.

Electron Transport Chain (ETC)

The electron transport chain (ETC) consists of four membrane-bound complexes of proteins that function as proton (H+) pumps.

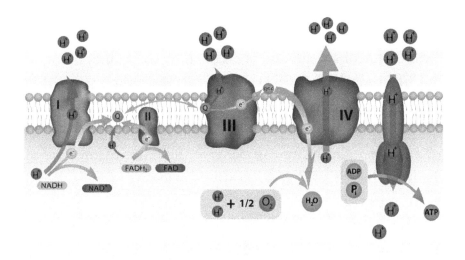

Electron transport chain for oxidative phosphorylation on the inner membrane of mitochondria.

Complex I and II pass electrons to CoQ10, which then passes them to Complex III. This in turn passes them to Cytochrome c. Cytochrome c passes electrons to Complex IV, which takes the electrons and two hydrogen ions (H+) created by the proton pumps and combines them with oxygen to form water in Complex V. Adenosine diphosphate (ADP) and phosphate combine in the presence of ATP synthase enzyme and form ATP. Complex V is like a turnstyle: a full rotation requires ten protons and releases three molecules of ATP.

Without oxygen the final destination for electrons is no longer available and cellular respiration stops. This happens with carbon monoxide poisoning where it displaces oxygen, causing the cells to die very quickly. Cyanide also kills by shutting down the ETC by inhibiting Complex IV, which stops the flow of electrons. The antidote is hydroxycobalamin (a form of vitamin B12), which reacts with cyanide to form cyanocobalamin and is excreted by the kidneys.

Unfortunately, the ETC is not 100% efficient so that some electrons escape the production line and leak into the matrix. They react with oxygen and form superoxide, a dangerous free radical that can damage the inner membrane of the mitochondria. This is known as oxidative stress and is a major cause of chronic diseases and aging.

It is interesting to note that many millions of years ago the mitochondria were originally another bacteria that "merged" or became symbiotic with the eukaryote cell. In exchange for food and protection from a high-oxygen environment, the bacteria will give their host cell extra energy for survival, resulting in advanced cells of plants, animals, and man.[1] In plants, the mitochondria became chloroplasts to take the sun's energy to turn it into ATP for plant cells.

Control of Oxidative Phosphorylation

Control over aerobic energy production is very important. There is constant fluctuation depending on the energy demands of the tissue. In order to respond efficiently, the mitochondria need to maintain on-site control by the mitochondrial DNA. To depend on the nuclear DNA would not be quick enough to meet sudden energy demand. When demand is high, electrons flow down the ETC rapidly and the proton gradient builds up quickly and more ATP is formed. When there is low demand, Complex V is forced to shut down and the electron flow slows and halts. There could also be a shortage of oxygen supply. That can stop the flow as well. When electrons back up, they can leak and create superoxide free radicals by combining prematurely to oxygen. So to avoid a wreck it's crucial to maintain a balanced oxidation-reduction on the ETC. If there is any shortage of a complex, the electrons back up and some will leave the line to form a free radical.

Free radicals are not all bad. They can control transcription factors, which alter gene activity to make more complexes for the ETC when needed, which is dependent on the level of ATP. They can also uncouple the electrons from the chain to produce body heat (ATP levels high). The trouble starts when too many free radicals are produced but not enough antioxidants to neutralize them.

The sum of all energy production in the entire body constitutes the basal metabolic rate of a person. The master thermostat of the energy furnaces in every cell is the thyroid gland. Basically, the thyroid hormones act on the mitochondria and control the speed of the entire oxidative metabolism and energy production. This increased energy in the form of ATP is used by the cells to increase their normal function.

ATP: Life's Energy Molecule

How do our cells utilize the energy molecule called ATP (adenosine triphosphate)? When a cell uses ATP for fuel, it breaks it down into ADP (adenosine diphosphate) and phosphate. When the phosphate bond is broken, energy is released for use. This process recycles by reattaching a phosphate molecule to the ADP into ATP, ready to be used again. This is a very efficient way to create energy rather than start from scratch.

There are one billion molecules of ATP in an average cell, and each molecule gets recycled about three times a minute. An average person has only about 1.75 ounces of ATP at any one time. Each mitochondrial ATP cycle can create about six hundred ATP molecules per second at maximum demand. This means that the 1.75 ounces of ATP are the equivalent of creating four hundred pounds of ATP in a day if there was no recycling[12]

Uncoupling the ETC for Heat

The ETC's proton gradient is not just used to produce energy; it can be uncoupled to release heat instead of ATP. The protons don't flow back through ATP synthase but through pores in the membrane called uncoupling proteins (UCP). This occurs in all warm-blooded animals. The advantages include adaptability to cold, muscle flexibility, and protection from mitochondrial damage by maintaining electron flow during low energy demand and less free radical formation.

The uncoupling is the source of non-shivering heat formation, which occurs predominantly in brown fat. Humans and mammals use muscles to shiver in intense cold or during exercise. Heat is also generated by the activity of other organs such as the brain and the heart.

In resting mammals, up to 25% of the proton gradient is lost as heat. Small animals and human infants need more brown fat, which has lots of mitochondria (hence the color) and UCP to generate heat. Brown fat is generally located in the neck, spine, and around the clavicles. The amount can increase with frequent cold exposure. It burns a large number of calories stored in white fat to produce heat. This is one way to help people prevent obesity and aging since there is less free radical damage. For example, the Inuit have a low incidence of degenerative diseases. Conversely, people of African descent don't need extra heat production, which means most of their ETC is for energy. They have a larger amount of free radical generation and higher chronic degenerative diseases. For these people, physical activity and exercise are critical to use up their ATP.[2]

NON-ENERGY FUNCTIONS

As if these functions are not enough, mitochondria are also involved in many essential non-energy functions. They contain enzymes for DNA/RNA and hemoglobin synthesis. They detoxify ammonia in the liver and synthesize sex hormones. They are involved in cholesterol and neurotransmitter metabolism, and free radical production (hydrogen peroxide) for immune cells. In addition, they store calcium for muscle contraction.

MITOCHONDRIAL BIOGENESIS

Just as our cells can eat up the low or non-functioning mitochondria (this process is called autophagy), it can also make new ones by division called mitochondrial fission or biogenesis. Two weak mitochondria can also fuse together to make a stronger one. Since there are multiple copies of mitochondrial DNA (mtDNA), the division isn't easy. The mtDNA can also be damaged by the free radicals and cause mutations, which can result in cell death. As you will see, we can increase the biogenesis process, which will increase our energy level.

You may wonder why mitochondria need their own DNA. Most of the genes are there to build the protein complexes of the ETC. Think of these protein complexes as the sub-stations or relay centers of an electricity generating plant that pass the electricity down the wires (the chain) to be consumed in the home (oxygen). Building more substations (complexes) allows more electricity to be passed to the home. So for our purposes here, these protein complexes give the mitochondria better control of its energy needs. If the free radicals signal for more complexes for the chain, the mtDNA that are in immediate proximity can respond to the demand rather than go through the nDNA in the nucleus. When mitochondria are not in control of their own destiny, the entire cell will have problems with energy production.

But not all the protein complexes are encoded in the mtDNA. They are a blend of proteins encoded by both mtDNA and nDNA. Only the crucial subunits are encoded by mtDNA, so they retain control of the assembly of new complexes. One important nDNA gene called PGC-1alpha is an important mediator of mitochondrial biogenesis and respiration.

When the cell divides, the separation of the mitochondria isn't necessarily equal. If there's a mixture of normal and dysfunctional mitochondria, the proportion may be uneven. If the new cell has more normal ones, it most likely will survive. The cell with more abnormal ones will die from inadequate energy.

MITOCHONDRIAL DNA MUTATIONS

Mutations in mtDNA may occur from free radical damage due to close proximity. If they lead to defective proteins in the subunits in the ETC, the rate of free radical leakage increases, which further damages mtDNA in a vicious cycle. This scenario is likely to happen because mtDNA doesn't have the protective histone proteins of nDNA, the repair mechanism is deficient, and there is no junk DNA.

There are two sets of genomes involved in making mitochondria function, mDNA (maternal) and nDNA (both parents), so inheritance patterns can range greatly. There are countless interactions between the two. The variation in mtDNA in the mother's eggs is surprisingly high.

When a cell divides, its mitochondria are distributed at random between the two daughter cells. One might inherit all the defective mitochondria, the other all healthy ones. The cell with all defective mitochondria will die by apoptosis. Each cell has different mitochondria with different mtDNA, which differ from organ to organ, leading to a vast range of possible disease symptoms. The onset of symptoms in this group of diseases can vary by decades, and even between siblings with identical genetic mitochondrial mutation.

AUTOPHAGY AND APOPTOSIS

What happens to the dead or dying mitochondria in the cell? They actually hinder overall energy production, so the cell would try to remove them in a process called mitophagy (controlled destruction). When an entire cell is senescent or dying, the entire cell would be removed by autophagy (self-eat). When they are eaten up, the cell function is improved. If the mechanism of apoptosis fails, a serious consequence is cancer. Apoptosis is critical for the integrity of the organism. The entire process of autophagy is controlled by the mitochondria!

Autophagy begins with the activation of certain membrane receptors and another organelle called the endoplasmic reticulum (ER). The mitochondrial apoptosis channel (mAC) is opened by certain stimuli, causing the outer membrane to become highly permeable, losing its electrical charge and proton gradient. This leads to a sudden burst in free radicals that oxidize various lipids (cardiolipin) of the inner membrane and bind to complex IV and shutting down the ETC.

This free radical burst also releases cytochrome c from the chain and form the "apoptosome," which then activates the enzymes of cell death, the caspases. They break down the cell in an orderly fashion. The cell shrinks and fragments but the organelles remain intact. Macrophages digest the fragments and recycle the components for reuse. In the human body, about ten billion cells are lost by apoptosis every day. This orderly process of apoptosis also occurs during embryonic development in humans. In some areas of the brain, more than 80% of the nerve cells disappear before birth. This kind of mass programmed death is necessary for the proper function of the organ.

CELL DANGER RESPONSE

Why do mitochondria lose their function? The answer lies in what's known as the cell danger response (CDR) first reported by Robert Naviaux[3]. It turns out that mitochondria's function is not just for energy production. It also senses danger from adverse conditions outside of the cell such as infections, inflammation, toxins, chemicals, etc. When these conditions are present, the mitochondria shut down the energy factory and alert the cell nucleus of these dangers. They shift out of energy production into cellular defense because the whole cell is threatened. Moreover, these two things are mutually exclusive: They can only do one of the two functions.

The mitochondria are also extremely sensitive to all sorts of environmental dangers such as EMF, ionizing radiation, chemicals in air or water, and heavy metals. They are like the canaries in the mine for a cell. Whatever the cause, the end result is the same, less energy production. If the outside attackers are strong and persistent, the mitochondria retract and eventually die. As the number and function decrease in a cell with high metabolism such as heart or brain, the function of these organs will be less than optimal and eventually symptoms start.

The attack on mitochondria can also come from within itself: the free radicals. It's like the exhaust in a car, a byproduct of its own metabolism. As more electrons are transported down the five complexes in the membrane, some escape and end up as free radicals (unpaired electron) also known as reactive oxygen species (ROS). These, in turn, can damage the mitochondrial membranes as well as other cellular structures including nuclear DNA. The end result is all the same: decreased energy production, structural damage, and eventually death.

CDR is the metabolic response that protects cells and host from harm. The first wave of danger signals consists of the release of metabolic intermediates like ATP, ADP, oxygen, and ROS After the danger has been eliminated, a choreographed sequence of anti-inflammatory and regenerative pathways is activated, which reverses the CDR. If the CDR persists, the body's entire metabolism and the gut microbiome are disturbed, multiple organ systems are impaired, the behavior is changed, and chronic disease results. An understanding of

CDR permits us to reconsider the causes of many chronic developmental, autoimmune, and degenerative disorders.

RESILIENCE THRESHOLD

Mitochondria have a third function beside energy and cell defense: They control your resilience threshold.[4] The more functional mitochondria you have, the greater your capacity to adapt to various stressors and a higher threshold for avoiding disease. The more dysfunctional and fragile mitochondria you have, the lower the threshold, and the easier to enter into stress overload and show symptoms. These symptoms include fatigue, sleep problems, post-exercise recovery difficulty, frequent eating to maintain energy, and brain symptoms like brain fog, anxiety, and depression.

In short, the health of your mitochondria reflects:
- Your energy level
- Your resilience to stressors
- Your resistance to disease
- Your aging and longevity

METABOLIC THEORY OF CANCER

The importance of the mitochondria is increasingly realized every year. The first breakthrough is the metabolic theory of cancer. This was first suggested by Dr. Otto Warburg in Germany in the early part of the twentieth century and more recently by Dr. Thomas Seyfried.[5] The conventional dogma of cancer is that it is caused by genetic mutations, which then causes mitochondrial failure. The metabolic theory is just the opposite in that the genetic changes are as a result of defective energy metabolism. The implications are earth shattering particularly in the treatment of cancer. So as long as your mitochondria remain healthy, your odds of developing cancer are small.

Cancer is such a dreaded disease that it claims the lives of more than 20,000 people daily. Part of the dread is from the treatments with significant side effects, including causing more cancers. If cancer can now be treated by treating mitochondrial dysfunction, this becomes a game changer. As you will see in later chapters, the functional treatment to boost mitochondrial energy production is without side effects. One example is following a ketogenic diet. Who could have imagined that a diet to lose weight turns out to prevent and fight cancer?

From this theory, recent research postulates that mitochondrial failure is the basis of all chronic degenerative diseases, from cardiovascular to neurodegenerative to metabolic like diabetes. Other conditions include ADD/ADHD, chronic fatigue syndrome, and fibromyalgia. Since the sex cells are high in mitochondria, infertility has a basis in mitochondrial dysfunction as well. In fact, the deteriorating mitochondrial function is at the crux of the aging process itself.

MITOCHONDRIAL THEORY OF AGING

When we are young, our mitochondria are abundant and working at an optimal level. As we age, mitochondria suffer wear and tear and lose their efficiency and eventually become non-functioning. According to a study by Linnane, Kovalenko, and Gingold, "muscle tissue of a ninety-year-old man contained 95% damaged mitochondria compared to no damage in a five-year-old." This translates into the vast difference in energy and activity level between those two age groups. The mitochondria lose number and change form. They show lower autophagy and biogenesis and increased apoptosis and mtDNA mutations.

The mitochondrial theory of aging was postulated by Anthony Linnane in the late 1980s.[6] This theory's main point is that the mitochondria is the main source of free radicals and that their accumulation is the cause of its dysfunction. Despite a repair mechanism called antioxidant enzymes that neutralize them, they become overwhelmed, and the mtDNA gets damaged. The mitochondria are the biologic clock controlling the aging process.

As cells lose energy production, they commit suicide called apoptosis. The latest research shows the mitochondria are controlling this process as well. With age, there is an accumulation of mutations in the control area of mtDNA that results in the death of the cell. If the mutation doesn't harm the mitochondrial function, it might result in free radical leakage. The defective mitochondria will signal their deficiency to the nucleus and switch off aerobic respiration toward anaerobic (not needing oxygen) fermentation, which produces much less energy. This then signals the cell to make new mitochondria to restore energy production. Therefore the number of mitochondria in a cell is constantly changing: amplify the least damaged ones (mitogenesis) and destroy the defective ones (mitophagy). They will be broken down and recycled into component parts.

With aging, our cells have more and more defective mitochondria, which still produce some level of energy but not low enough for mitophagy. The cell and its mitochondria then reach a new equilibrium by adapting their behavior. When enough cells are in this condition, we start noticing easy fatigue and decreased endurance. After years in this state, the cells eventually run out of healthy mitochondria to replicate and only defective ones are replicated, and at some point they are given the signal to commit apoptosis, ending in a steady loss of tissue function and ultimately death.

Research by Frank Shallenberger, M.D. indicates that nearly 50% of people under age forty have early onset mitochondrial dysfunction (EOMD) and virtually everyone over forty has it to a very significant level. I see mitochondrial problems in teenagers and even kids. Between the ages of twenty and forty, and between forty and seventy, your mitochondrial capacity and number get cut in half. So at seventy, your mitochondria are a quarter of the number and function of age twenty! This is the course of normal aging, not taking into account the increasing levels of toxic load we're all exposed to. EOMD is reversible if you catch it before diseases are diagnosed.

On top of the natural decline of aging, there is also a lack of mitochondrial stimulation, which is more important. Our modern lifestyle leads to very little hormesis, which is a temporary stressor that increases resistance to other stressors and elevates the resilience threshold. Keep in mind that the stressor is of short duration, and a period of rest and regeneration is necessary to prevent harm.

Another recent measure of aging is the telomere length. These are the caps at the ends of chromosomes much like the ones on a shoelace. A little is lost with each cell division and when they are too short, the cell dies by apoptosis. Telomere length is thus a measure of the declining function of the cell. Cancer cells, however, continue to divide without limit, perhaps by induced telomerase activity. Studies have shown mitochondrial dysfunction plays a role in inducing telomere shortening and therefore a shortened lifespan of the cell.

Mitochondrial metabolism is tied to our food and caloric consumption. If we reduce consumption, fewer electrons pass through the ETC and there is less leakage of free radicals and vice versa. This is why obesity is linked to numerous chronic diseases. There is still much to learn here, but new research shows the cell is better at repairing damaged mDNA than we thought previously, so the cell should be able to keep going for much longer than we know now.

If we could slow the rate of free radical leakage from the mitochondria, we could delay the onset of degenerative diseases and perhaps eliminate them. Keeping mitochondria healthy and free of mutations is the key to address chronic degenerative diseases and aging at this time. This opens up a whole new world of prevention rather than disease treatment. We will discuss this issue in the next chapter.

CHAPTER SUMMARY

1. Mitochondria are structures within the cell that produce energy (ATP) from food and oxygen. There are several hundred to thousands depending on the energy demand of the tissue.

2. The more energy is produced, the more free radicals are produced that can damage the mitochondria.

3. Energy production stops where there are dangers to the cell in the form of adverse conditions (cell danger response).

4. Mitochondria control the orderly process of cell death (autophagy).

5. Biogenesis is the making of new mitochondria when there is the need.

6. Mitochondrial dysfunction is the cause of chronic diseases, aging, and cancer.

CHAPTER TWO

PREVENT MITOCHONDRIAL DAMAGE

So far we have discussed the mitochondria's function on a cellular level. We've seen that they are the energy generators of the cell that makes ATP, which is needed for all cellular functions. We've also seen how this function can be shut off when it senses the cell is under dangerous conditions such as infections, inflammation, toxins, etc. Free radicals are formed in the process of energy production that can damage mitochondria. They can also undergo mDNA mutations that may affect their function and end in chronic diseases, cancer, and aging. What can be done to slow or reverse the damage? The first and most crucial step is to remove chemicals and toxins from our bodies. This will allow the nutrients to enter the cell and repair the damage by making new mitochondria. We will explore this topic in this chapter.

CHEMICALS, POLLUTANTS, AND TOXINS

The mitochondria are sensitive to attack from both outside and inside the cell. The external attacks can come from the environment, food, and water. We're all drowning in a sea of chemicals in the air. These include car exhaust, water from the tap, and chemicals and preservatives in food. Now a new danger is the rampant use of pesticides like glyphosate (Roundup), which has been demonstrated to paralyze the electron transport chain and increase free radicals in mitochondria.[7]

We have to be aware of the commercial personal hygiene products that we all use. They are loaded with chemicals, preservatives, and perfumes. It is the same in our commercial processed foods that come in boxes and containers. If you read the labels, they will show a long list of chemicals, colorants, artificial flavors and preservatives.

Then there are the thousands of medications that are consumed, many of which damage the mitochondria and cause side effects. This includes all psychotropics, analgesics, statins, and many antibiotics. Many of the side effects of chemotherapy are from the toxic effect on the mitochondria of non-cancer cells. Radiation also damages the mitochondria as well as DNA.

Heavy metals constitute a major group of toxins. These include mercury, aluminum, lead, cadmium, thallium, lead, and arsenic. They are characterized by high molecular weight and density and are poisonous in low concentrations. In today's world, they are increasing exponentially and their widespread use leads to a significant percentage of patients we see in functional medicine. They are widespread in the environment and foods.

After exposure, toxins tend to have an affinity for certain tissues, predominantly brain and fat. They're not evenly distributed once inside the cell but tend to be drawn into the mitochondria and concentrated there. The effect is generally an inhibition of the ETC, but in the case of arsenic, the effect could also be on mtDNA. Tin dispels the charge of the outer membrane. Thallium is ten times more toxic than mercury. The overall effect of heavy metals is to prevent nutrients from entering the mitochondria to make energy. They must be removed from tissues by a detoxification program before the mitochondria can recover.

Other chemicals or medications exert their effect by increasing free radical production. As we mentioned before, free radicals are molecules with unpaired electrons and have a negative charge. They are highly reactive with other molecules since they need to pair the charge to become stable. The result is oxidative damage to lipids, DNA, proteins, and carbohydrates leading to cell damage. That's why we need antioxidants to quench the excess before they damage the cell.

FREE RADICALS AND ANTIOXIDANTS

Free radicals are the toxins internally produced within mitochondria. There are different types of free radicals. One of the most dangerous is a free radical of oxygen called reactive oxygen species (ROS). There are also reactive nitrogen species (NOS), hydroxyl radicals, superoxides, and hydrogen peroxide. They are derived from normal metabolic functions or from external sources such as exposure to X-rays, ozone, cigarette smoke, air pollutants, and industrial chemicals and drugs. Internally generated sources include high mitochondrial metabolism, inflammation, strenuous exercise, lack of oxygen, and ischemia (poor blood flow). Chronic free radical damage results in free radical diseases associated with aging such as cancer and atherosclerosis.

More recent research shows the free radicals are not all bad. They also have beneficial functions such as killing microbes (hydrogen peroxide) and signaling the nucleus to make more components of the ECT. It is the balance of oxidants and anti-oxidants that determine cell damage and disease formation. If the balance is chronically unfavorable, a condition known as oxidative stress results. The injured tissues produce increased radical-generating enzymes that activate phago-cytes, the release of copper and free iron from storage, and disruption of the ECT. This results in more ROS and less energy production.

The development of cancer and side effects of radiation and chemotherapy are examples of this imbalance. Other examples are diabetes, macular degeneration, and neurodegen-erative diseases such as Parkinson's and Alzheimer's disease. In fact, oxidative stress is implicated in all inflammatory dis-eases, ischemic diseases, and alcoholism.

Antioxidants can decrease oxidative stress by scavenging ROS or inhibiting cell proliferation. They are molecules that can donate an electron to the unpaired electron of free radicals and neutralize them before they do harm. Some antioxidants such as glutathione, ubiquinol, and uric acid, are produced during normal metabolism in the body. Others come from fruits and vegetables in the diet or in supplement form. We will discuss these in detail in later chapters.

The principal dietary antioxidants are vitamin C, vitamin E, and β-carotene, or vitamin A. Our body cannot manufacture them, so they must be supplied in the diet. For example, vitamin A found in carrots is protective against skin cancer that is from excess sunlight. Vitamin C, one of the most powerful antioxidants, can fight cancer, inflammation, and infections. Vitamin E plays a role in the stimulation of the immune system. The combination of all three vitamins gives an additive effect and has the highest reduction in developing cardiac disease and cancer.

Free radicals are implicated in the aging process itself either indirectly or directly. Direct damage to DNA or the accumulation of cellular and functional damage to other cell structures such as mitochondria play a role. Reduction of free radicals or decreasing their rate of production may delay aging. The optimal intake of antioxidant nutrients may contribute to a higher quality of life in the elderly and may even prolong life span.

During normal oxidative phosphorylation, 0.4–4.0% of all the oxygen consumed is converted in the mitochondria to superoxide free radicals. The cell can transform superoxide to hydrogen peroxide by superoxide dismutase. Hydrogen peroxide can then be converted to water by glutathione peroxidase. If this enzyme is not adequate, as it was for me, then damage accumulates in the mitochondria.

There is no excessive free radical production when there is low fuel (food) as in starvation, or when there is plenty of fuel and high activity and oxygen like a well-fed athlete. The problem arises in a well-fed sedentary person because there is high ATP production but little need and the ETCs become backed up with excess electrons. Now there is a high rate of free radical leakage that exceeds the antioxidant defense system. Once this process crosses a threshold, pores in the outer membrane open up and initiate the first steps of cellular suicide (apoptosis).

STRESS

Now let's look at another major cause of mitochondrial dysfunction: stress.[8] Psychological and social stress, negative emotional states, and psychiatric disorders have been shown to negatively impact the mitochondria. Recent discoveries implicate the mitochondria in two major ways: as a target of stress and as mediator of stress. Rats subjected to stress showed mitochondrial dysfunction and increased free radical production and damage to lipid membranes. There was also depletion of glutathione, the body's most important detoxification compound.

High stress levels cause shallow breathing and less oxygen delivered to the cells. Stress raises the hormone cortisol, which breaks down skeletal muscle that contains the highest concentration of mitochondria. It can interfere with methylation and regulation of our feel-good neurotransmitters, serotonin and dopamine. In short, to optimize mitochondrial function, you must include anti-stress measures.

INFECTIONS

Bacterial, fungal, and viral infections can also adversely affect the mitochondria. Earlier we had discussed the cell danger response where mitochondria can shut down the energy factory in order to fight invading pathogens. This includes its ability to turn on our immune system or induce programmed cell death. Bacteria can manipulate cell organelles like the mitochondria to hide from our immune system that destroys them. Since the mitochondria are involved in the regulation of the innate immune response and energy production, they are a primary target for destruction by the pathogens.

Viruses either induce or inhibit various mitochondrial processes in specific ways so that they can replicate in the cell. Viruses like herpes simplex 1 deplete the host mitochondrial DNA and some, like human immunodeficiency virus, hijack the host mitochondrial proteins from functioning in the cell. The hallmark of viral infections is profound fatigue from the shut down of the energy factory.

INFLAMMATION

Inflammation in the body of any cause can also trigger mitochondrial dysfunction. Experimental evidence supports this association, particularly in the brain. Inflammatory mediators called cytokines produced by activated immune cells will trigger a shut down of the energy production and increase ROS as part of the cell danger response. This process may ultimately result in cell death. If severely damaged mitochondria are not removed by mitophagy, they can release their contents into the cell and increase inflammation with more pain, swelling, and redness in the affected areas.

SEDENTARY LIFESTYLE

Not moving throughout the day is a major problem in industrialized countries where too many people have desk jobs and sit in front of a computer all day. They walk a few steps to their cars and drive home, only to eat fast food or take out. They spend the rest of the evening sitting in front of the television or more computer time on social media. This takes a toll on our musculoskeletal system, which can weaken and atrophy, depleting more mitochondria. This lifestyle slows down our basal metabolism and a slower rate of eliminating the free radicals leading to oxidative stress. Basic movements such as doing house chores and taking a walk around the block after eating have been shown to increase metabolism and enhance the longevity of people living in the blue zones (areas of the world with the longest average life expectancy). They don't work out in health clubs, but they all do chores, work in the fields, and spend more time outdoors. We will examine the role of exercise and the mitochondria in Chapter Six.

EXCESS FOOD CONSUMPTION AND ALCOHOL

Overeating along with not moving is doubly bad on the mitochondria. The metabolism of excess food without the utilization of ATP produces abundant free radicals and oxidative stress. If the diet is a typical Western one, with abundant fried foods in vegetable oil, processed food with preservatives and chemicals, there is even greater oxidative stress. Large quantities of meat and carbohydrates, along with inadequate digestive enzymes and slowed transit time, allow fermentation by gut bacteria and bloating, inflammation, pain, and cramping. Overgrowth of bacteria in small intestines is known as SIBO, and dysbiosis in the colon. The toxins from bacterial fermentation further damage the mitochondria, which can cause fibromyalgia and chronic fatigue syndrome.

If alcohol is consumed in excess with food, the mitochondria are further compromised. In fact, few other toxic substances destroy mitochondria as quickly as alcohol, which predisposes you to the development of chronic degenerative diseases including diabetes, obesity, heart disease, and dementia. These have all been linked to mitochondrial dysfunction.

ELECTROMAGNETIC FIELDS (EMF)

Not to be confused with PEMF, EMF consists of electromagnetic radiation from cell phones and towers, microwaves, appliances, and Internet routers. The higher-frequency EMFs, which include X-rays and gamma rays, are in the ionizing radiation part of the spectrum and can damage DNA and cells directly. The low-to-mid-frequency EMFs are non-ionizing and include household appliances and wireless telecommunication devices such as wireless tablets and laptops, and microwaves ovens. Most Wi-Fi networks operate at frequencies similar to cell phones, typically 2.5GHz and recently 5.0GHz.

Mitochondria are semiconductive, and the process of creating energy (oxidative phosphorylation) is electrical; therefore EMF affects the mitochondria. Studies have shown cell phones near the genital area will reduce sperm quality and testosterone levels. Since sperm consumes high levels of energy for its motility, exposure to EMF can have an 85% increase in free radicals. EMF can also affect the myelin sheath insulating your nerves, which slow down nerve conduction and increase the risk of developing multiple sclerosis. EMF increases blood sugar because mitochondria are not metabolizing the sugar into energy efficiently. EMFs cause a danger response in molds, causing them to turn aggressive and produce more mycotoxins.

Artificial EMF can damage the mitochondria in as few as three hours. Changes can be seen in the form as swelling, cavitations, and broken cristae (folds of the inner membrane). There is increased lipid peroxidation and free radical formation. The calcium ion channels controlled by mitochondria become open, and the increased intracellular calcium leads to termination of ATP formation and ends in apoptosis. Basically, EMF causes oxidative stress with increased ROS and mtDNA mutations and decreased antioxidants.

Protect yourself from EMF by keeping your cell phone away from the body, not in your pants pocket or in your bra. Distance is your friend with EMF; the intensity drops by the square of the distance. Use a headset or a speakerphone. Turn off the Internet router at night and don't keep electronic equipment near you when you sleep. Use a grounding mat indoors, or better yet, ground yourself outdoors or at the beach where EMF is lowest. Maintain a set circadian rhythm and get restful sleep. Magnesium supplementation can help block the calcium ion channel opening.

In summary, our mitochondria in every cell are not only energy producers but also are highly sensitive to external and internal toxins, inflammation, and infections. They turn off the normal energy production (cell danger response) and over time become damaged by the excessive release of free radicals. The stress that most people live under, along with the sad American diet (SAD) and sedentary lifestyle, all add up to progressive mitochondrial dysfunction and death leading to all the most common chronic diseases of today. It is not a pretty picture unless we start to reverse it. In the next chapter, you will see how nutrition and diet can help reverse mitochondrial dysfunction.

CHAPTER SUMMARY

1. To optimize mitochondrial function, we have to avoid exposure to chemicals, pollutants, and toxins (including biotoxins), and heavy metals.

2. Avoid medications like psychotropics, statins, and antibiotics.
3. Reduce stress: emotional, physical, and dietary.
4. Treat infections and inflammation including autoimmunity.
5. Avoid caloric excess, alcohol, and a sedentary lifestyle.
6. Avoid EMF exposure that damages mitochondria.

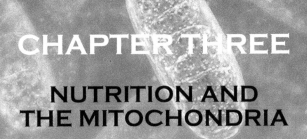

CHAPTER THREE

NUTRITION AND THE MITOCHONDRIA

To maintain healthy mitochondria we first need to eliminate harmful substances that damage them. We then feed them the food nutrients that nourish them to optimize function. These are both the right mix of macronutrients (fat, protein, and carbohydrates), which are burned as fuel with oxygen, and micronutrients such as minerals and phytonutrients. This is our topic for this chapter.

ELIMINATION DIET

We need to eliminate all foods that cause inflammation, infections, and toxins such as pesticides. Genetically modified foods (GMO) also must be removed since they have been modified to resist pesticide use. All these factors cause leaky gut by altering the microbiome, which is the community of micro-organisms (bacteria, fungi, and virus) that live in a particular environment like the gut. We have seen how the increased permeability of the gut lining causes a reactive inflammation that may spread throughout the body leading to autoimmunity. Inflammation and infection in the body cause the mitochondria to shut down energy production as part of the cell danger response.

We must start by eliminating the following food groups for four to six weeks:

- Sugar and artificial sweeteners
- Dairy products (milk, cheese, yogurt, ice cream)
- Gluten (wheat, barley, rye) and all grains
- Alcohol
- Beans and legumes (soy, peanuts, and cashews)
- Fruits and vegetables high in fermentable carbohydrates (FODMAP): onions, broccoli, cabbage, apples, and pears.
- Eggs
- Vegetable oils and trans fats in processed foods

You may be surprised by the FODMAP items since they are healthy for us.[9] This is for those who experience gas and bloating after meals. You may lack the enzymes to break down and absorb the sugars that feed bacteria, which leads to fermentation, especially in those with an imbalance in the microbiome known as dysbiosis or small intestinal bacterial overgrowth (SIBO). The fermentable carbohydrates (fructans, galactans, lactose, and polyols) can cause explosive gas and diarrhea. If you have these symptoms, you need to eliminate these items:

- Beans, soy products including soy sauce
- Onions, garlic, green onions
- Broccoli and cauliflower, cabbage, etc. (Brassica family)
- Apples and pears
- Peaches, plums, and nectarines

After the elimination phase, you should feel better with fewer digestive issues, fatigue, or pain. Now you are ready to reintroduce them back one at a time to see if symptoms return. Keep a food diary to keep things straight. Wait three to four days after each reintroduction before the next one. If symptoms return, eliminate that food.

Start with the most healthy vegetables, beans, and eggs (the most perfect protein). The rest of the list should be avoided permanently, especially if you have mitochondrial issues and chronic diseases.

Dairy contains lactose (a fermentable carbohydrate) to which many adults are intolerant because of a lack of lactase enzyme. It also contains casein and whey that many have trouble digesting.

Gluten is a family of proteins that are present in all forms of grains. The most common is alpha-gliadin present in wheat, barley, rye, spelt, kamut, and triticale, all of which are very difficult to digest. Some people have a genetic disposition to react to them called gluten sensitivity and celiac disease. Other grains contain other forms of gluten protein such as avenin in oats and oryzenin in rice but in lower amounts.

Some may be sensitive to these as well. So just avoiding the classic gluten (alpha-gliadin) foods will not eliminate all symptoms for this reason.

Sugar we know now is the main culprit in all the chronic metabolic diseases, not cholesterol. Even though it is the quickest energy source for the body, excess amounts can damage the mitochondria and produce inflammation and free radicals (oxidative stress). It also paralyzes the immune cells for several hours. High levels can trigger reactions with proteins called advanced glycation end products (AGE) that cause abnormal function in many organs. If you're addicted to sugar, the best alternatives are stevia and monk fruit.

Beans are very healthy and serve as a protein source in vegetarians. However, they contain galactans, a fermentable carbohydrate. They also contain lectins, but proper cooking and canning remove them. In a grain-free diet, beans and sweet potatoes are good substitutes.

Soy products also contain fermentable carbohydrates, are GMO, and contain pesticides. Organic is the way to go as it is with fruits and vegetables. Pesticides like glyphosate have been shown to produce a leaky gut.

Eliminating food sensitivities and allergies will have a major impact on your health. They sap your energy and increase inflammation and oxidative stress that are all related to mitochondrial dysfunction.

KETOGENIC DIET[10]

The ketogenic diet is one that is low in carbohydrates (10%), moderate in proteins (20%), and high in fat (70%). Mitochondria can burn fuel either as glucose from carbohydrates or fatty acids from fat. When we consume fat and not glucose, it forces the liver to make ketones from fat, which is burned more efficiently in the mitochondria and produce fewer free radicals. It is like burning a cleaner fuel in a car with less exhaust. Because ketones result in more energy and lower inflammation, the brain is sharper and you lose weight, especially belly fat. Unfortunately, most people are used to a high carbohydrate diet (70%–80% of calories), which is addictive, makes insulin spike, which then brings down the glucose too low and results in hunger and cravings a few hours after eating.

In contrast, when the body is keto-adapted to run on ketones, the blood sugar is low and stable, so no insulin spikes and no cravings or hunger occur. So we have to change the diet where the carbohydrates come mainly from plants but not starchy roots like potatoes. The protein should be from grass-fed, clean animals. The good types of fat are olive, avocado, and coconut oils as well as butter from grass-fed cows. Medium-chain triglycerides (MCT) oil is a portion of the coconut oil that can easily be turned into ketones.

It is not a good idea to eat a lot of bacon and other processed meats if they're not from clean animals and are chemically processed. Eating too much protein will also convert into carbohydrates and kick you out of ketosis. Desserts can be made from stevia or monk fruit as sweeteners and will keep you in ketosis.

During the keto-adaptive phase, which may last two to four weeks, your body is recalibrating to burn fat instead of glucose. You may feel minor side effects that should go away quickly. These include keto breath, flu-like symptoms, muscle cramps, bowel changes, etc. You must be well hydrated and add some sea salt and magnesium to the water.

There are two main types of ketogenic diet: standard and cyclical. The standard is to remain in ketosis permanently. Your carbs are limited to 20–50 grams per day and protein around 1.0 grams/kg of body weight. In the cyclical, you periodically consume higher amounts of carbs to come out of ketosis. You can cycle one or two days a week or once a month. People often tolerate this better because there is less stress reaction on the body since it does not think you are in a starvation state.

INTERMITTENT FASTING

The ketogenic diet is even more effective when coupled with some form of intermittent fasting. The benefits of fasting are numerous:
- Heal your leaky gut and improve microbiome
- Reduce inflammation
- Improve insulin and other hormone sensitivity
- Increase growth hormone
- Burn more fat and lose weight
- Stimulates cellular autophagy and DNA repair

- Protection from chronic diseases
- Longevity

When I personally combined keto diet with intermittent fasting, the weight came off effortlessly, particularly the stubborn belly and visceral fat around organs.

The benefits of calorie restriction again relate to the mitochondria. Fewer calories mean less fuel (as electrons) entering the ETC, with a corresponding reduction in free radical formation. Calorie restriction could extend lifespan by up to 60% in animal studies, making a human lifespan of 130–150 years a possibility. Such restriction has been shown to be effective in disease prevention as well as to stay biologically younger longer. They delayed most major diseases such as cancers, heart disease, diabetes, hypertension, and autoimmunity. Furthermore, calorie restriction does not need to be started at an early age to reap benefits. This is good news for people who don't begin to think about health and longevity until their fifties and sixties!

INTERMITTENT FASTING STRATEGIES

When you first begin, start with a shorter fast of twelve hours and build up gradually as your body adapts. An example is to finish dinner by 7 p.m. and eat breakfast the next morning at 7 a.m. This allows the liver to cleanse the blood from the gut and allow rest and digest to take place. You sleep better and heal faster. You then build up to fourteen or sixteen hours of fasting with a liquid breakfast of a beverage with some added

MCT oil to tide you over to lunch. A strong fast is 16–18 hours fasting on a daily basis. This has the most benefit for most people as it did for me. During your eating window of six hours, you can eat two meals plus a snack without calorie restriction. You continue until you have achieved your weight goal or improvement of your health condition.

On a weekly basis, you can do a 24-hour fast once a week of your choice. A longer fast increases autophagy. Some people prefer this to a daily 16-hour fast because of work schedules. You can also combine daily intermittent fasting, one 24-hour fast, and a cyclic ketogenic diet. An example is intermittent fasting Monday through Friday, a higher carb re-feed day on Saturday, and a 24-hour fast from Saturday night to Sunday night dinnertime. It is best to refrain from binge eating after the fasting day. Those with adrenal fatigue or exhaustion may need more carbohydrates, so the carb re-feed day or two may work better.

Research shows if you fast for five days per month for three months in a row, there is improved cell regeneration, decreased risk factors for chronic diseases, and anti-aging effects. During fast days, make sure to manage your stress levels and replenish salt and minerals.

FASTING MIMICKING DIET (FMD)

Very recently there is a new diet called ProLon developed by Dr. Valter Longo at USC that mimics a total fast for five days, yet you can still eat light pre-formed meals each day of around 800 calories. It's like fasting with training wheels and

I recommend it to patients who want to kickstart a ketogenic diet. You will lose three to five pounds and still have normal activities and even light exercise. The advantage is greater autophagy and production of stem cells to regenerate tissues. Done over three successive months, the benefits remain over time. It is the only patented anti-aging method so far in this country.

EXOGENOUS KETONE

Exogenous ketones made of beta hydroxybutyrates is a supplement to get into ketosis quicker or when your body has dips in ketone levels. It is useful also to preserve your muscle from breaking down if you have prolonged or intense exercise. Some use it when they just ate some carbs that take them out of ketosis. There's no point to use these if you stay in ketosis. Using a ketone meter can be helpful for this purpose.

MITOCHONDRIA-BOOSTING DIET

Epigenetics is the study of changing gene expression without changing the genes that occur in response to environmental factors. Nutrigenomics is when those factors are food nutrients. This is how powerful food can be on our health. No medication can come close to doing this.

So what can you eat to boost your general and mitochondrial health? The answer is whole natural organic foods that are not packaged or processed. This means free-range, grass-fed/grass-finished meat, cage-free organic eggs, organic fruits and vegetables, tree nuts, seeds, and wild fish. The best fish with low mercury are wild Alaskan salmon, cod, herring, anchovies, sardines, and mackerel. Tuna once a week is acceptable and there are tuna that have been tested for mercury. A limited amount of whole grains within the guidelines of a ketogenic diet is good if you have no sensitivity.

The best foods for the mitochondria are those that have high antioxidants since free radicals damage them. They are the basic vitamins A, B, C, D, and E. The above foods have them in abundance. The phytonutrients that give color to fruits and vegetables are also rich in antioxidants and minerals. Examples are carotenoids in yellow and orange vegetables, lutein in green leafy vegetables, and anthocyanin in purple and red ones. Vegetables make the body more alkaline, which helps the ETC in mitochondria, whereas acidic environment signals cell danger response. There should be no additives, dyes, or preservatives that may harm the mitochondria.

Most American diets contain excessive animal proteins, often processed or cured in sulfites like luncheon meat. A small quantity of clean protein (one gram per kg of body weight) is good to strengthen muscle, which has a high quantity of mitochondria. Older people find it hard to digest the protein because they don't have enough digestive enzymes and acid in the stomach. Taking betaine HCl and pancreatic enzymes can help.

Eating slowly and chewing your food twenty times is important for digestion. You want to sit and relax and be grateful before a meal. Even something as basic as sitting down to eat can improve digestion because cortisol is released standing! These simple steps all stimulate the parasympathetic system to rest and digest rather than the sympathetic system of fight or flight. In the next chapter, we will discuss the main supplements you can take before or with your diet plan.

CHAPTER SUMMARY

1. Reduce gut inflammation with an elimination diet to exclude sugar, dairy, gluten, soy, alcohol, legumes, eggs, fermentable fruits, and vegetables.
2. A ketogenic diet allows mitochondria to burn fuel more efficiently with fewer free radicals that cause oxidative stress.
3. Intermittent fasting strategies stimulate cellular and mitochondrial autophagy (housecleaning) and biogenesis (form new mitochondria).
4. A mitochondria-boosting diet consists of organic whole foods with balanced macronutrients and micronutrients (antioxidants, vitamins, minerals).
5. Eat slowly, chew well, and be relaxed in order to stimulate the parasympathetic system that comes from proper rest and digestion.

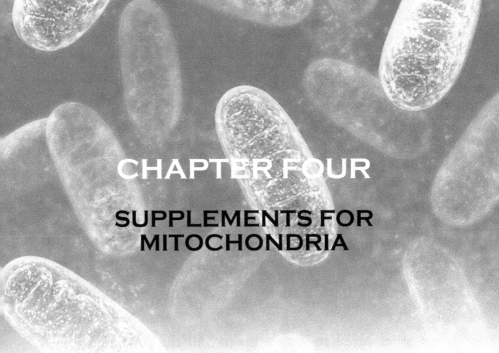

CHAPTER FOUR

SUPPLEMENTS FOR MITOCHONDRIA

I believe your diet is always the best way to nourish your body and mitochondria in the long term. Supplements are used as a temporary bridge while you learn to eat a healthier diet and live a better lifestyle. They can quickly reboot a chronic mitochondrial dysfunction once the toxins, chemicals, and unhealthy lifestyle factors have been removed.

MULTIVITAMIN AND MINERAL FORMULA

Whatever your current health condition, everyone should take a multi-vitamin and mineral supplement. These include vitamins A, B, C, D, E, K and magnesium, calcium, potassium, selenium, chromium, and zinc. These are all essential nutrients that support the body and prevent mitochondrial damage leading to disease and aging. It is very hard to obtain all these nutrients from our food today due to soil depletion and non-organic farming practice. Many people have malabsorption of fat-soluble vitamins due to medications and low secretion stomach acid and enzymes. A multivitamin is the best health insurance for the price.

Go for the highest quality of multi-vitamin and not quantity. Make sure it contains natural folate instead of synthetic folic acid. Folic acid competes for the same receptor site as natural folate, and conversion to the active form 5-MTHF is slow, leaving unconverted folate, which is a health risk. It is particularly important for pregnant mothers to have the folate form.

Another problem is that up to half the population has a genetic mutation in the MTHFR gene, which affects methylation. The result is an elevated homocysteine level, which can damage the cardiovascular system. For these people, the 5-MTHF form is recommended. By the way, this gene mutation called a single nucleotide polymorphism (SNP) is easily tested with an oral swab test.

Multivitamin and minerals formulas come in a multi-pack, which is both convenient and provides adequate dosage. Some may contain fish oil and antioxidants as well. The once-daily pack forms the foundation of a supplement program regardless of the specific condition.

GLUTATHIONE (GSH)

Glutathione is the most important antioxidant and detoxifier in the body. It consists of three amino acids: glutamine, glycine, and cysteine and is made in the liver. It has many important functions, including:

- DNA synthesis and repair
- Support immune function
- Absorb free radicals
- Regenerate vitamins C and E
- Transport mercury out of the brain
- Assist with cell death (apoptosis)
- Decrease inflammation and infections
- Decrease cancer, degenerative disease, and aging
- Enhance athletic and mental performance
- Detoxify chemicals, pesticides, EMF, radiation, alcohol
- Improve insulin sensitivity
- Treat autism spectrum disorders

Glutathione is found in meat, fish, poultry and cruciferous vegetables (broccoli, Brussels sprouts, cauliflower, kale, etc.). Spinach, avocados, asparagus, and okra are some of the richest dietary sources.

Allium vegetables such as garlic, shallots, and onions rich in sulfur compounds can raise glutathione through cysteine. Folate (vitamin B9) also boosts glutathione production. Whey protein is another good source of cysteine.

Some supplements activate natural glutathione production in the body. N-acetyl-cysteine (NAC) is the direct precursor form to glutathione and is much less expensive. Vitamin C helps renew oxidized glutathione back to the active form. Just 500 mg for thirteen weeks leads to an 18%–47% increase in intracellular glutathione. Selenium is a cofactor for the production of glutathione and can be found in fish and Brazil nuts. Milk thistle supplements are another way to boost glutathione levels naturally. Turmeric and curcumin (extract form) have the ability to increase glutathione levels.

Adequate sleep and regular exercise are also vital to maintain a healthy glutathione level. A combination of both cardio and weight training will do the most to increase glutathione. Overtraining without adequate nutrition and rest can decrease its level. Finally, alcohol can decrease glutathione levels in the liver, brain, pancreas, and lungs. Most people don't realize the small airways of the lungs have a high concentration of glutathione, which is depleted by 80%–90% by chronic alcohol use.

Glutathione supplement has absorption problems. The best form is liposomal where it is enrobed in a lipid bilayer to increase absorption. The dose is 300 mg per day.

CoQ10

CoQ10 is a vitamin-like molecule naturally present in every single cell in the body and essential to life. It is part of the ETC and is a rate-limiting step in energy production in mitochondria. Its synthesis requires an amino acid tyrosine, eight vitamins, and trace minerals. Like glutathione, we produce less CoQ10 as we age. So its decline is associated with the aging process. Since we get very little from our food, supplementation becomes increasingly important as we get older. It is an antioxidant, a membrane stabilizer, and regulates gene expression and apoptosis. CoQ10 also has anti-inflammatory, redox modulatory, and neuroprotective effects.

CoQ10 is part of the ETC positioned right after Complex I where most of the free radicals are produced. It can even take free radicals and put their electrons back into the ETC to make energy. So it is critically positioned to soak up free radicals right at the site of production and thereby protect the mDNA, membranes, and other enzymes. It is also found in other cell organelles functioning as an antioxidant.

Congestive heart failure and cardiomyopathy are conditions where the heart muscle is weak from mitochondrial dysfunction. They lead to lack of oxygenation and further energy decline. New studies using high doses of the absorbable form is proving CoQ10 to be one of the most important nutrients for mitochondrial health for these conditions.

CoQ10 also lowers blood pressure by neutralizing peroxynitrite free radicals, so there is more nitric oxide for dilation of blood vessels and reduce platelet stickiness. These free radicals can damage the blood vessel lining. Ubiquinol can keep the LDL cholesterol in a reduced state, which prevents it from doing harm in your body. For this reason, ubiquinol could be a superior alternative to statins to protect against heart disease.

Absorption of this large fat-soluble molecule is also challenging. Oil-based formulations in soft gels are much better absorbed. The water-dispersible liposomal form is better as is the reduced form ubiquinol instead of ubiquinone. This conversion slows down past age twenty-five, so ubiquinol is by far the superior form for bioavailability.

Many medications deplete CoQ10, the primary one being statins for lowering cholesterol. The side effects of statins are felt to be lower energy production in the mitochondria. Taking ubiquinol is a must if you're on a statin. Beta-blockers for hypertension are another group of drugs that deplete CoQ10 and accounts for the fatigue. CoQ10 may also decrease the effectiveness of warfarin, a blood thinner but not for other classes of thinners.

Ubiquinol can also be used as an anti-aging product. Many experts believe optimizing mitochondria is one of the most powerful strategies to extend your life. It has been shown that our oxidative stress increases significantly with age. This supplement can decrease degenerative diseases and extend lifespan. Mice studies showed the ubiquinol group at the equivalent age of 90–100 in human years ran around like teenage mice while the control group was near death. It was able to bring 80% of children with Down's syndrome back to normal oxidative levels within a month. Ubiquinol has a positive effect on:

- Inflammatory processes
- Septic shock
- Cardiac arrest recovery
- Stroke recovery
- Periodontal disease
- Neurologic diseases: Down's, Parkinson's, Huntington's, and Alzheimer's disease

The recommended dosage of CoQ10 100–200 mg per day in a healthy individual taking statins but could be doubled in mitochondrial dysfunction or failure. Its safety profile has been very high even at very high doses with no interactions with medications. For ubiquinol, the dose is 100 mg per day. When you first start taking CoQ10, start out at 200–300 mg a day, and after three weeks, go down to 100 mg maintenance per day. Divided doses, of up to two or three times a day, are best. Athletes and people with severe congestive heart failure should take 300–600 mg/day. Neurologic conditions require 600–3000 mg per day.

There is a new form of CoQ10 called MitoQ. This molecule is positively charged while mitochondria are negatively charged, so it is electrostatically pulled into the mitochondria between 800 and 1200 times greater than regular CoQ10. Good results are reported for chronic fatigue syndrome and MS and Parkinson's disease. The dose here is 10–20 mg per day.

PYRROLOQUINOLINE QUINONE (PQQ)

This new product is the only one that can generate new mitochondria (mitogenesis). In the past, it was believed that only strenuous exercise or calorie restriction can induce it. It can also protect nerve cells and promote nerve growth. PQQ is capable of catalyzing continuous redox (oxidation and reduction reactions) for thousands of cycles. It is widely distributed in animal and plant tissues.

PQQ appears to act through PGC-1 alpha, which is a transcriptional coactivator that regulates genes involved in energy metabolism. It is associated with a reduction in free radicals and protection against mitochondrial toxins. PQQ has been shown to activate other transcription factors such as NRF2 that lead to increased mitochondrial biogenesis. Another beneficial effect is as a cofactor in one of the subunits of Complex I of the ETC, the main producer of free radicals. In humans, PQQ improves reproduction, growth and development, and immune function. It reduces the damage from ischemia-reperfusion, heart attacks, and stroke.

Evidence now points PQQ as an unidentified essential B vitamin. Mice eating a PQQ-free diet had impaired reproductive, growth, and immune function. These mice had abnormally small mitochondria that didn't function properly. It also activates a key enzyme in collagen production, hence the abnormal skin and connective tissue of these mice.

A supplement of oral PQQ (20 mg per day) improved short-term memory, attention and concentration, and processing speed. The effect is enhanced with CoQ10 since it is also part of the ETC. Luckily, PQQ is present in high concentration in cocoa powder, hence the benefits of dark chocolate. It's also in parsley, green tea, and green pepper.

FREE FORM AMINO ACIDS

This is a combination of the essential amino acids that we can't make in the body in a powder form. For mitochondrial failure or dysfunction, it is necessary to give these amino acids in a single high-dose bolus of nine grams, mixed in water or juice, on an empty stomach. This may be given twice a day in severe cases. The idea is to saturate the mitochondria with all the amino acids they need to synthesize the subunits of the ETC complexes and thereby kickstart the energy production. I generally add 1000 mg of tryptophan since it is the rate-limiting step in protein synthesis. The free amino acids are easily absorbed compared to eating protein like meat where only about a third is actually absorbed.

Supplementing with essential amino acids is also important in the elderly. As we age, our absorption of proteins declines considerably so that by the time we're eighty years old, we've reduced our muscle mass by half (muscle wasting is called sarcopenia). It's worse if you are inflamed or are under chronic stress, which can put you in a catabolic (tissue breakdown) state. Mitochondria make up 10% of our muscle mass, so with less muscle, you end up with less energy. The elderly need to consume more proteins, and the most digestible form is eggs. Free form amino acids, particularly branched-chained ones (BCAA), are particularly usable by the muscle. In athletes, it also helps muscle recovery after exercise. If you're vegetarian or vegan, supplementation is vital to your mitochondrial health.

MAGNESIUM

Magnesium is often a neglected mineral and most people in the world are deficient for many reasons: the soil is depleted, the use of water softeners, a high intake of calcium and caffeine, and use of antacids and proton pump inhibitors. This is bad news because magnesium is a critical cofactor in more than three hundred biochemical reactions in the body, including the production and binding with ATP, making it more stable and usable by the body.

Without magnesium, our muscles can't relax. For the smooth muscles of blood vessels, a deficiency leads to vaso-constriction and less oxygen delivery and less energy production in the mitochondria. So this deficiency translates into high blood pressure, ischemic heart disease, congestive heart failure, angina, atherosclerosis, and stroke. It's also linked to asthma, diabetes, osteoporosis, PMS, and colon cancer. Within the Krebs cycle, magnesium is an essential cofactor. It is also essential for brain function like memory and cognition. All these conditions are linked to mitochondrial function.

Dosage in mitochondrial failure is 400–600 mg spaced throughout the day. The chelated (combined to amino acids) form is better absorbed. The citrate or oxide form can relieve constipation. Magnesium threonate helps anxiety and brain function. Taken at night, it can help sleep by relaxing the muscles. Magnesium even helps set and regulate cell energy over the circadian cycle.

LIPID REPLACEMENT THERAPY (LRT) AND OMEGA 3 FATTY ACIDS (DHA)

Omega 3 fatty acids (specifically DHA) and phosphatidyl-choline are two nutrients essential for the protection of the cellular and mitochondrial membrane function and repair. Since the ETC is located on the inner membrane, its proper maintenance is key to its function. It helps fight inflammation and maintain brain structure. It can significantly reduce moderate to severe chronic fatigue and restore mitochondrial function in a matter of weeks.

You can obtain DHA from fish oil 1000–2000 mg per day or better yet, krill oil which can be absorbed directly by your brain without additional processing. It also has approximately forty-eight times more antioxidants than fish oil. Astaxanthin, the compound that makes salmon red, also protects mitochondria from oxidative stress and increases resilience. They can be combined together and taken with a fatty meal or MCT oil for better absorption.

Lipid replacement therapy can be obtained in a product called NTFactor, a supplement combining phosphatidylcholine, probiotics, growth media, and antioxidants. This product has been shown to be effective for chemotherapy-induced fatigue, nausea and vomiting, and diarrhea by reversing the membrane damage caused by free radicals. The dosage is one to three tablet three times a day for mild to severe fatigue. It also comes as a chewable.

L-CARNITINE

L-carnitine is the main ingredient to shuttle fat through the mitochondrial membrane where it can be burned as fuel for energy. Fat is the main energy source, constituting 60%–70%. If you're deficient in L-carnitine from a genetic variant, you can't burn your fat and so this becomes one of the reasons why you can't lose weight no matter what you do. You can see this deficiency in the first three markers of the organic acids test.

Another important role of L-carnitine is clearing lactic acid buildup. This is a by-product of anaerobic metabolism where there is not enough oxygen for aerobic metabolism or when energy demand is suddenly too great. You feel the lactic acid burn in the muscles during strenuous exercise along with fatigue. I experienced this at the height of my leg stiffness, and just a small chore like washing dishes or grocery shopping can leave me fatigued. L-carnitine is useful for peripheral vascular disease, angina, congestive heart failure, arrhythmia, fatty liver, diabetes, exercise intolerance, and weight loss.

L-carnitine in the diet comes mainly from animal-based products and is negligible in plants. Approximately 25% comes from our own internal production, which accounts for up to 90% for vegetarians. Dosage is 500 mg per day.

CREATINE MONOHYDRATE

Creatine monohydrate is a stable and bioavailable form of creatine often used by body builders for muscle enhancement and performance. Ninety-five percent of the body's creatine is stored in the muscles in the form of phosphocreatine, which can donate a phosphate to ADP to make our energy currency ATP. More ATP in the muscle is very useful in high-intensity interval training so you can maintain high performance longer. It raises anabolic hormones such as IGF-1 and testosterone, and reduces protein breakdown, resulting in greater muscle mass.

A creatine supplement can also increase phosphocreatine in the brain, which may improve function and prevent degenerative diseases. In older adults with sarcopenia, it can dramatically increase muscle mass in conjunction with weight training.

Start with a loading dose of 20 grams per day in four divided doses for the first week. Then take 3–5 grams per day as maintenance. If you don't load, it will take you three to four weeks to maximize your stores.

ALPHA LIPOIC ACID (ALA)

Lipoic acid is a cofactor for the enzymes catalyzing the final stages of glycolysis so it can enter the Krebs cycle. A deficiency can be seen in the organic acids test with elevated carbohydrate markers.

It has the unique ability to function as both a water- and fat-soluble antioxidant. ALA has an important role in the production of glutathione. It is targeted to the mitochondria while other antioxidants can't be concentrated to a useful level.

ALA modulates the energy carrier NAD in its free and reduced forms. Excess NADH leads to free radical damage. Even more concerning is that excess NADH, in the absence of sufficient numbers of ETCs, causes the mitochondria to become backed up with excessive electrons, which react with oxygen leading to the formation of superoxide radicals. It can even influence the aging process through activation of genes called sirtuins, which are anti-aging. ALA can increase NAD+ while a decrease of NADH turns on the sirtuin genes.

NICOTINAMIDE RIBOSIDE

Nicotinamide riboside is a form of vitamin B3 (niacin), which is a precursor to NAD^+ and plays an important role in energy production in the mitochondria. It is present in all cells but declines 50% from ages forty to sixty. It further declines from caloric excess, alcohol, and stress. Scientists think this decline is part of the natural aging process. Taking this supplement can increase NAD^+ by 50% after eight weeks. You will feel more energetic and have greater resilience to stress. Dosage is two capsules of 150 mg.

D-RIBOSE

D-ribose is a simple five-carbon sugar, which is a structural component of DNA and RNA and ATP. Supplemental D-ribose given to ischemic hearts could wake up the dormant areas and have faster energy recovery. It has been used in recovery from cardiac surgery, congestive heart failure, and restored energy to depleted skeletal muscles. Athletes use it to improve performance. Those with fibromyalgia also report improvement in pain and stiffness. These symptoms are due to a build-up of lactic acid from anaerobic glycolysis rather than aerobic. It is useful for those using a ketogenic diet. Doses as low as 500 mg could be beneficial, but standard dosages are 3–5 grams per day. Increase the dose until relief of symptoms is noted, as it is safe even at large doses. It does not impact blood glucose or insulin levels.

CANNABINOIDS AND ENDOCANNABINOID SYSTEM

The endocannabinoid system is present in most living organisms including man. It is considered the master regulator of homeostasis in the body. We produce our own cannabinoid compounds called endocannabinoids as opposed to phytocannabinoids found in plants. The two main compounds in the cannabis plant are cannabidiol (CBD) and tetrahydrocannabinol (THC). The THC receptors are mainly in the brain and nervous system and CBD receptors are mainly in the body. They often show opposite effects under different situations and dosages.

In 2012, French scientists discovered that mitochondria contained cannabinoid receptors on their membranes.[11] Both THC and CBD can affect mitochondria. No doubt homeostasis involving energy production are controlled by this system. They accomplish this by a biphasic dose-response curve meaning two opposite responses are possible depending on the dose. Low-dose THC tends to increase mitochondrial activity, while higher doses tend to decrease it. The context in which the signal is produced (what else is going on in the cell and mitochondria) is also taken into consideration.

This type of biphasic response is similar to that of the free-radical signal. There's evidence of cross-talk between the

ECS and the free-radical system. These interactions in the two systems can be stimulatory and inhibitory, depending on the cell context, and therefore acts to fine-tune homeostasis. However, abnormalities in either system could undermine the stability of both systems and contribute to dysfunction and disease states.

Research on the brain shows THC can inhibit the formation of amyloid plaques by increasing mitochondrial function. CBD has been shown to induce mitochondrial biogenesis and reverse memory loss in animals. CBD can protect against brain injury by regulating intracellular calcium. An imbalance of calcium in the mitochondria might drive Alzheimer's disease, hence the connection between the two.

These two cannabinoids are just the two major classes, but there are many more minor compounds as well as terpenes. As in all botanical medicines, the whole is greater than the parts and we must study the full spectrum of beneficial compounds. Since we have receptors on all body systems, the effects of cannabinoids are far-reaching and so far we have only scratched the surface.

POLYPHENOLS AND FLAVONOIDS

Over the last decades, an increasing number of studies have shown that dietary polyphenols can regulate mitochondrial redox status, and in some cases prevent or delay disease progression. One study looked at the role of four dietary polyphenols—resveratrol, curcumin, epigallocatechin-3-gallate

(EGCG), and quercetin—in molecular pathways regulated by mitochondria and their potential impact in human health. It showed that the polyphenols improve mitochondrial functions. The mechanisms underlying the polyphenols' beneficial effects include decreasing oxidative stress, regulation of mitochondrial metabolism, biogenesis, and apoptosis. The understanding of the chemical-biological interactions of dietary polyphenols with mitochondria may have a major impact on the treatment of mitochondrial dysfunction.

According to Dr. Barry Sears, we should be getting at least 2000 mg of polyphenols per day but most get between 200 mg and 1000 mg. Coffee is the largest source of polyphenols in the Western diet. The benefits of coffee are highest at five cups per day, regular or decaf. Each cup has 200–500 mg of polyphenols, followed by tea, chocolate, and red wine. You still need to supplement with a mixture of polyphenols from different fruit extracts, resveratrol, and pterostilbene. One unique product is coffee fruit extract containing a mix of polyphenols shown to increase BDNF for brain health.

Flavonoids are the largest group of polyphenols and are responsible for the colors in fruits and vegetables. Polyphenols and flavonoids are not transported in a free form. They are bound to either sulfur or glucuronic acid and are inactive. But at sites of inflammation or infection, the cells release an enzyme called glucuronidase. This liberates them and allows them to enter the cell's mitochondria and protect them from free radical damage. They also activate genomes that allow the mitochondria to function more efficiently. They not only nourish our cells but also our gut microbiome. Polyphenol levels can be seen in the general bacteria section of the organic acids test.

SULFORAPHANE

This is a sulfur-containing compound found in the Brassica family of vegetables such as broccoli, kale, cauliflower, cabbage, etc. It is beneficial to mitochondria by inducing apoptosis in many cancer cell lines while protective against oxidative stress in normal cells. It also promotes mitochondrial biogenesis in normal cells. As a supplement, take 10 mg daily with a bite of raw radish or cruciferous vegetables to provide the living enzyme in your gut to activate the supplement. You can also eat raw broccoli sprouts, which have the highest sulforaphane content.

KETOPRIME

This supplement is very powerful for rapidly boosting your mitochondria to clear brain fog especially resulting from excess glutamate, i.e., MSG. It contains oxaloacetic acid (OAA), which is the final step in the Krebs cycle that accepts acetyl-CoA from the metabolism of glucose, protein, or fat. The more OAA you have, the more it can metabolize sugar and fat. Ketoprime mimics the mitochondrial effect of fasting, which turns on your sirtuin genes that make you live longer. It also increases NAD+ necessary to make energy and protects mitochondria from environmental toxins and free radicals. Being water-soluble, it can cross the blood-brain barrier for its brain effects.

Dosage is 100 mg sublingual (under the tongue), one or more times per day as needed, up to ten times. You can use it before workouts, or anytime you feel symptoms of mitochondrial dysfunction (headaches, fatigue, brain fog).

BERBERINE

Berberine is an alkaloid, which tends to be stronger in their effect than the flavonoids. Flavonoids are neutralized fairly quickly in the body by binding to glucuronic acid or sulfur. Alkaloids circulate in two to three forms and therefore tend to be stronger. Like PQQ, berberine benefits mitochondrial function and is a powerful AMPK activator that increases longevity. Dosage is 1500 mg in divided doses.

MELATONIN

Melatonin, a hormone of the pineal gland in the brain, has been shown to possess numerous protective actions. Its relationship to mitochondria is more profound than previously believed. Melatonin is also formed in the mitochondria, which also contain melatonin receptors. Melatonin is not only synthesized in the pineal gland but in numerous and perhaps almost all organs. The quantities of extra-pineal melatonin exceed those in the pineal gland by many times but are usually not released into the blood stream for general circulation. The mitochondria-protecting actions of melatonin are diverse and may be considered a defense weapon. Melatonin decreases nitric oxide free radical (NO) formation in the brain, thereby reducing its damaging effects. It also reduces electron leakage by regulating electron flow down the ETC and by preventing the opening of mitochondrial membrane pores through which electrons can leak out. It scavenges free radicals, increases levels of antioxidants such as reduced glutathione (GSH), and can also prevent apoptosis.

ADAPTOGENS/CORDYCEPS MUSHROOMS

Adaptogens are natural herbal products that work in the cells to normalize their function and maintain homeostasis (balance) in response to stress. One powerful adaptogen is Rhodiola rosea, which enhances mitochondrial energy production and is a powerful antioxidant. Dosage is 200–400 mg in the morning.

Another favorite adaptogen of mine is the ayurvedic herb ashwagandha (Withania somnifera). It is very effective for stress, anxiety, and depression, and has been shown to reduce cortisol level. It can reduce blood sugar, fight cancer and inflammation, and boost testosterone. It has been shown to increase muscle mass (which increases mitochondria) and reduce body fat. On top of all that, it lowers cholesterol and increases brain function and memory! Not bad for one herb. Dosage for a standardized root extract is 500 mg capsule once or twice per day.

Cordyceps mushrooms have been prized in China for centuries. It is considered a "superfood" in that it is an adaptogen that can slow aging, prevent disease, and boost energy. It is anti-inflammatory, antioxidant, and anti-cancer. Cordyceps can boost brain function, enhance memory, and extend longevity. The animal model showed cordyceps increased the activity of antioxidants like superoxide dismutase (SOD) and glutathione. This mushroom can boost athletic performance by increasing ATP since it contains adenosine, a nucleic acid that is needed to make ATP. It is also a natural treatment for infertility and impotence.

B VITAMINS

The B vitamins undoubtedly have the greatest direct impact on cell metabolism and energy production either as a cofactor or a precursor in a reaction. Eight out of twelve are essential (that is, they can't be made by the body): B1, 2, 3, 5, 7, 9, and 12. They're all water soluble, so there is no accumulation in body fat.

Vitamin B1 (thiamine) functions in carbohydrate metabolism to convert pyruvate to acetyl-CoA to enter the Krebs cycle. It also serves to maintain the nervous system, memory, and heart muscle. A true deficiency causes beriberi, a circulatory-system disease that is seen only in alcoholics. A high carbohydrate diet may require more thiamine. This can be seen in the organic acids test under the carbohydrate section.

Vitamin B2 (riboflavin) is a major component of the cofactor in Complex I of the ETC and FAD in Complex II.

FAD shuttles electrons from the Krebs cycle to the ETC. If there is a Complex I deficiency, riboflavin can help bypass this by channeling electrons to Complex II.

Vitamin B3 (niacinamide and niacin) are the main forms in supplements. Niacin is a safe and inexpensive treatment for high LDL and low HDL cholesterol. It is the precursor to NAD+, which is essential to mitochondrial function. NAD+ is involved in regulating sirtuin gene function in aging (sirtuins are proteins that help regulate cellular health). Nicotinamide riboside is the most efficient precursor of NAD+/NADH. Vitamin B3 is used to treat neuropathies and neurodegenerative diseases, diabetes, cancers, and inflammation.

Vitamin B5 (pantothenic acid or pantethine) has a very important role in the body as a precursor of coenzyme A (CoA), which is essential for the metabolism of carbohydrates, proteins, and fats through aerobic metabolism in the mitochondria. It is needed in the synthesis of steroid hormones and melatonin. It is important for the synthesis of the neurotransmitter acetylcholine critical for memory, and heme, a component of hemoglobin that carries oxygen.

Vitamin B6 (pyridoxine) is necessary for the proper function of more than seventy different enzymes of energy metabolism. It is also involved in the synthesis of neurotransmitters in the brain for mood and hemoglobin synthesis.

Vitamin B12 (cobalamin) is the only vitamin containing a mineral: cobalt. It is found in many foods such as fish, shellfish, meat, eggs, and dairy but is negligible in vegetarian sources. B12's main function is supplying methyl groups for protein and DNA synthesis. For the mitochondria, B12 is involved in the generation of S-adenosyl methionine (SAMe), which is a part of various protein subunits that make up the complexes in the ETC. The absorption of vitamin B12 requires intrinsic factor made by parietal cells in the stomach. An autoimmune attack on these cells leads to pernicious anemia. Vitamin B12 injections are required for this condition.

Vitamin D deficiency has also been found to affect mitochondrial function particularly in human muscle and must be corrected (because most people are deficient in vitamin D, and 25% of all mitochondria reside in the muscle, so it affects overall energy). Sunlight with its UV light is best to activate vitamin D3. It works even better if you pair it with vitamin K2 and vitamin A.

IRON

Iron is an essential mineral and an important component of proteins in oxygen transport and metabolism. Heme, the functional form of iron, is synthesized by the mitochondria. It makes up hemoglobin and myoglobin in skeletal muscle. It is an essential component of proteins within the complexes of the ETC. When heme metabolism is disrupted, the result is mitochondrial decay, oxidative stress, and iron accumulation, all hallmarks of aging.

Biosynthesis of heme requires multiple B vitamins, biotin, alpha lipoic acid, and the minerals zinc, iron, and copper. If any component is deficient, heme synthesis is affected. Iron deficiency anemia is the number one anemia worldwide, particularly in women of childbearing ages. Their lack of energy is due to a reduction in the number of ETC complexes in operation.

Do not supplement with iron unless it is based on a blood test. Too much iron can increase the free-radical and lead to a number of neurodegenerative conditions such as Parkinson's and Alzheimer's, cancer, and can even result in death.

RESVERATROL AND PTEROSTILBENE

The benefits from resveratrol and pterostilbene are not due to their being antioxidants but instead, are due to their ability to turn on or off certain genes (gene expression) through epigenetics. Resveratrol of the French Paradox fame has received interest for its anti-aging benefits. It is closely related to a compound called pterostilbene found in blueberries and grapes. They have similar structures and function and work in a synergistic fashion on gene expression.

Both products have the ability to mimic many of the beneficial effects of calorie restriction by regulating genes involved in the development of a variety of age-related diseases. Their complementary action might help prevent cancers and diabetes and promote longevity. Many of these benefits relate back to the mitochondria.

In the next chapter, we will examine all forms of lifestyle habits and hormesis that can increase the number and function of mitochondria.

CHAPTER SUMMARY

1. Mitochondrial function depends on multiple B vitamins and minerals, so a multivitamin and mineral formula is a must.
2. Glutathione and CoQ10 are two critical components of energy production.
3. Antioxidants are important to neutralize free radicals from oxidative stress.
4. Free form amino acids improve energy production by synthesizing protein components of the ETC.

CHAPTER FIVE

LIFESTYLE AND HORMESIS

HORMESIS/BIOHACKING: DEFINITIONS

Hormesis refers to a bi-phasic response to an environmental stimulus characterized as a low-dose beneficial response and a high-dose harmful or toxic effect. This is often applicable to the mitochondria, where a low or short stimulus produces a beneficial strengthening to the body but is harmful at high intensity or prolonged stimulation. This makes sense if you understand how the ETC works. Low intensity and duration pushes the electrons through the chain or makes the mitochondria divide to meet the demand. High intensity produces too many free radicals because electrons are held up on the ETC by slower rate steps.

Biohacking is the art and science of changing your environment around and inside you so you have full control over your own biology in order to maximize your full potential. It was popularized by Dave Asprey, CEO of Bulletproof, who started experimenting on himself to find shortcuts to better energy, productivity, and longevity. There are many biohacks in his book *Headstrong,*[12] which I highly recommend for those who want to maximize mitochondrial function, delay aging, and prolong longevity. I and some of my patients share this interest, and functional medicine is the perfect vehicle for this goal.

Our Paleolithic-era ancestors experienced much more hormesis compared to the modern world. They spent most of the day hunting and gathering with periods of fasting due to food scarcity and exposure to heat and cold. Now we live in an age of anti-hormesis where little movement or exercise is required, food is plentiful, we can eat empty calories anytime, and we live in a climate-controlled environment where we never need to sweat or shiver. These conditions all lead to mitochondrial atrophy and dysfunction. No wonder we have such an epidemic of chronic degenerative diseases! Hormesis is the basis of good health, disease resistance, and longevity.

The mechanisms of hormesis are multiple. One is that stress creates a transient burst of reactive oxygen species (ROS), which stimulates our cellular antioxidant defense system to grow stronger. Another is increased autophagy, which stimulates the cells to repair and rebuild new parts that function like new. This process can double the number of mitochondria and double your energy capacity. Another mechanism is the production of heat shock proteins (HSP) following hormetic stressors, which aid in the proper folding of intracellular proteins. The result is muscle growth, mental clarity, and better mood.

Research shows us that hormesis is the key to maintaining healthy mitochondrial levels. It's possible to have strong, abundant mitochondria as we grow older. The natural aging decline in mitochondria doesn't have to happen if we're exposed regularly to hormetic stressors.

EXERCISE/HIIT

Exercise and physical activity are probably the most important for mitochondrial health. It is the classic hormesis in that short and low to moderate intensity are beneficial while exhaustive and prolonged ultramarathons are detrimental by producing excessive free radicals and pro-inflammatory mediators that damage muscles and other organs. The damage is worse if there is no recovery time. Moderate regular exercise leads to fewer cardiovascular diseases, cancer, diabetes, and mortality.

It seems paradoxical that moderate exercise, which induces increased free radicals, does not damage the mitochondria. The increased energy demand results in fission and biogenesis through signaling from the relative abundance of AMP versus ATP by the free radicals themselves. With frequent moderate exercise, the number of mitochondria per cell has increased, and each one has more ETC. The end result is more spare capacity of energy at rest with fewer free radicals. We become more resilient to sudden stresses without going into anaerobic respiration.

Physical activity also uses up the ATP produced by the extra mitochondria, so there is no backlog of energy and production of free radicals. So it's the free radicals in combination with insufficient ATP that trigger biogenesis. This is the link between exercise and improvements in cardiovascular, cognitive, mood, and musculoskeletal health. Longevity is also increased and premature death is avoided.

Aerobic exercise can increase the number of mitochondria by 50% in six weeks. The intensity has to be at least half of your maximum capacity and sustained for twenty minutes three to four times a week. It also modifies gene expression for brain-derived neurotrophic factor (BDNF), which increases neurons in the hippocampus responsible for memory. BDNF also stimulates neuroplasticity, which is the connectivity of the neurons to adapt to stress. Pregnant rats that exercised improved mitogenesis even in their offspring.

Resistance exercises like weight lifting don't seem to have the same effects on their mitochondria. It does, however, have a great effect on preventing age-related muscle wasting (sarcopenia) in the elderly.

High-intensity interval training (HIIT) is characterized by repeated bursts of intense exercise of short duration (thirty seconds to one minute) alternating with light exercise for recovery of equal duration. This can be done on the treadmill or other equipment. These bursts can be done about seven to ten times. Compared to long aerobic workouts of half to one hour, HIIT can be completed in ten minutes. It is also much better in increasing muscle mitochondria and endurance.

OXYGEN AND BREATHING

We are rarely aware of our breathing. Yet we know that oxygen is the final electron carrier in the mitochondrial ETC to form water. In fact, that's the reason we need to breathe. But most people are stressed and breathe in a very shallow and quick way that does not oxygenate well. Chest breathing only uses the top of the lungs, which is the smallest area and is poorly vascularized.

We need to breathe from the belly by contracting the diaphragm and expanding the abdomen. This opens the large bases of the lungs, which has the most blood circulation. Practice by placing one hand over the chest and the other on the belly. Breathe through your nose only. The belly needs to move in and out much more than the chest. Breathe in for a count of four, then out for six or eight to let all the air out. This will slow the rate down but each breath is deeper. Practice this every time you are stressed; you will immediately feel more relaxed. Practice whenever you can and soon it becomes a habit.

There is another breathing technique called Buteyko popularized by Patrick McKeown. You breathe slowly (around eight breaths per minute at rest) and gently through the nose using belly breathing. This releases nitrous oxide, which opens the blood vessels and 20% more oxygen is delivered to the tissues. The slow quiet breathing also has a calming effect. The rate should be so slow that you feel slight oxygen deprivation. This allows the carbon dioxide to build up in the blood, which allows a greater release of oxygen from its carrier hemoglobin. This technique is very good to train kids with asthma and chronic sinusitis to stop mouth breathing, which can deform their oral cavity. Buteyko breathing has also been shown to reduce oxidative stress.

HYPOXIA

Long-term hypoxia (oxygen deprivation) will lead to cell damage and death from excessive free radical formation. However, if we limit oxygen for short periods of time (intermittent hypoxia training) it's possible to increase the efficiency of oxygen intake and reduce oxidative stress damage. This form of hormetic stress on the mitochondria causes them to either grow stronger or undergo cell death (apoptosis). It also helps build more mitochondria. Like classic hormesis, it trains the strong and eliminates the weak. It also increases the production of BDNF, which grows new neurons. You become more resilient to low oxygen like airplanes, high altitudes, and stress.

Because of air pollution, the oxygen level of our city air has been dropping even more so than the increase in carbon dioxide. The air quality inside our homes and offices are often worse than outside. Gyms can be even worse with lots of people exercising in an enclosed space often without adequate ventilation.

Professional athletes take advantage of this hack to train in high altitudes or do intermittent hypoxic training. This consists of intervals of breathing low oxygen air through an air mask, alternating with intervals of breathing regular air. The body becomes more efficient at delivering oxygen to the tissue, so it boosts athletic performance and eliminates weak mitochondria to grow new ones.

A free hypoxic exercise is the walking breath holds. You exhale and hold. Count the number of paces you can do before you need to breathe. Breathe until you return to normal breathing. Repeat four to twelve times. You can also do the breath-holding pranayama exercise. Take thirty to fifty short breaths of rapid in and out through the nose, then breathe out all the air and hold your breath as long as possible.

STRESS REDUCTION

Mental stress is very detrimental to the function of mitochondria either directly or indirectly. They can sense stress and negative energy in the body through electromagnetic fields. Indirectly, mental stress elevates cortisol, which has a catabolic effect on the lining of the gut leading to leaky gut and inflammation, which is a cause of oxidative stress. Also, try listening to relaxing music while taking a warm bath with Epsom salt before bed. Aromatherapy with lavender is also very effective along with a cup of herbal tea.

Laughter is a great stress reducer and has been underutilized. It reduces stress hormones cortisol, adrenalin, and noradrenalin. It increases endorphins and serotonin, the feel-good neurotransmitter. It boosts immunity and blood flow to the organs. A good belly laugh increases lung capacity and oxygen delivery to the cells, especially when stressed and breathing is shallow. Best of all, you can learn laughing exercises to become happy. The laugh should be loud, deep and in multiple bursts with the head tilted up. It is also infectious, and doing it with others becomes powerful.

MEDITATION

The best solution to mental or emotional stress is meditation. This is no longer a woo-woo fad; it is becoming mainstream and essential for stressed-out people from all walks of life. There is now abundant research that shows how beneficial meditation is for your brain. It literally changes the structure of the brain, from deeper folds of the surface correlated with intelligence, to a thicker corpus callosum, which connects the left and right brain. You will have both logical and creative problem-solving skills. Meditation also leads to a significantly reduced level of stress hormones and inflammation. The result is calm focus, emotional stability, empathy with others, and improved relationships.

Of course, meditation has a positive impact on your mitochondria. Coupled with breath work, the boost is even greater. How does meditation affect the rest of the body? Probably through the mitochondria since they are present in all body systems. They sense the environment around them whether physical or emotional and tailor their energy production accordingly. The calming effect of meditation can thereby increase energy production.

Personally, meditation is best combined with spiritual mindfulness and connection to God or the divine. I visualize being connected to God by light which travels through me and returns back to Him with each breath. In this light are love, abundance, and health down to the mitochondrial level. It's as if the entire body is recharged by this divine energy. You can visualize areas of pain disappearing as you push the energy to that area. Use this time to manifest the life and health you want to have. Just fifteen minutes first thing in the morning sets the tone for the whole day instead of letting your emails dictate your day!

SLEEP

Sleep is also critical to the mitochondria. In Chapter Five we saw how melatonin is involved with the ETC and energy production. It's the only antioxidant to act very specifically to reduce oxidative stress on the mitochondria. Sleep is literally making more energy for you while reducing oxidative stress. And it's free!

Melatonin is involved in the circadian rhythm for our bodies. We know this is really critical for all body functions, particularly the adrenal glands. As you recall, the production of cortisol follows a predictable diurnal pattern that peaks in the morning, then drops off through the day, and is lowest at bedtime, allowing melatonin to rise at night. We all know the effect of jet lag when we travel and nothing feels right.

The quality of our sleep is more important than quantity. We need to have enough deep sleep in order for the brain to flush out accumulated junk like amyloid through the glymphatic system.[13] This is a newly discovered system of lymphatic channels around blood vessels that drain cerebrospinal fluid through the brain tissue. They are controlled by the glial cells, hence the term glymphatic. The brain shrinks down to half size to create these lymphatic channels that drain out the waste. It's literally like a toilet flush that washes out neurotoxins and drains into the bloodstream. This flush is one of the main functions of sleep and is so vital that we spend one-third of our lives sleeping. Some people boast of how little sleep they can get away with. This is foolish thing because trying to get by on only four or five hours of sleep night after night amounts to dooming yourself to brain fog, disrupted circadian rhythm, hormonal imbalance, gut problems, cravings, and obesity. Humans need seven to eight hours of sleep per night. This claim has now become a documented fact.

The glymphatic drainage system is active only during sleep because it requires a lot of energy. If it happened during the day, there would not be enough energy to do your usual daytime activities. It's only during sleep with low-energy usage elsewhere that it can be done, all powered by the mitochondria. The more efficiently they work, the shorter the time for sleep and the better the quality of sleep. You'll wake up refreshed and mentally sharp, thanks to those hard-working mitochondria.

Sleep hygiene is critical to get to sleep at the proper time (ideally no later than ten o'clock). Too much blue light from TVs and computers and other stimuli like working late into the night will turn off melatonin production and prevent sleep. So use blue light blockers on the screens or glasses and turn them off an hour before bedtime. Don't use white LED lights at night and switch to red light. Avoid alcohol, drugs, and caffeine in the evening. Don't read in bed even if it relaxing because you want to associate bed with sleep. If you can't fall asleep after twenty minutes, get up and do something else until you feel sleepy. Do not exercise within an hour or two before bed.

We have discussed stress reduction techniques like breath work and meditation, bath, music, massage, etc. These can all be helpful if you have trouble falling asleep. It's vital that you follow a daily routine to establish a circadian rhythm of sleep and wake cycles. If you have to travel, use melatonin to reset the rhythm to local time and follow the same sleep hygiene you normally practice.

CIRCADIAN RHYTHM

All life on Earth is in tune with the daily rhythm of light and dark. Most organisms including humans have their metabolic, physiologic, and behavioral processes synchronized to a 24-hour clock. New research has discovered that the circadian rhythm is a primary factor for our general health, body composition, and energy levels. It is a major contributor to most degenerative diseases like obesity, diabetes, heart disease, and cancer.

Disrupted circadian rhythm has been shown to:
- Contribute to inflammation and weakened immune system
- Increase stress hormones
- Predispose to cancer and accelerate tumor growth
- Increase neurodegenerative diseases
- Seriously impair memory

- Accelerate aging
- Decrease energy levels and daytime sleepiness
- Increase the overall risk of dying from any cause
- Decreased autophagy (cell breakdown) and biogenesis (new mitochondria formation).

There are three main factors that dictate our circadian rhythm:
1. Light and dark
2. Movement
3. Nutrients

Modern civilization is now 24/7. We live life indoors with artificial light and minimal sun exposure. We are exposed to blue light from our electronic screens late into the night, which keeps our brain awake. We don't move as much as our ancestors did. Our nutrients are often deficient from processed and fast foods. The net effect is the disruption of autophagy and massively decreased energy levels and quality of life.

One simple trick to increase autophagy is to decrease the concentration of the amino acid leucine in the blood. You can do this by drinking water 8–12 ounces first thing in the morning at least forty-five minutes before breakfast. Autophagy is also increased during fasting, so try to prolong the fasting window as long as possible.

Our current eating habits are very contrary to establishing a stable diurnal eating pattern. Most people eat throughout the day and evening and fast only during sleep. They eat the largest meal in the evenings after 6 p.m. or just before bedtime. The majority of calories were consumed between meals as snacks. There is also significant variation in meal timing from weekdays to weekends, which can amount to what can fairly be called metabolic jetlag. Our bodies crave regularity in meal times, activity times, and sleep. Any disturbance from the routine will throw off the circadian rhythm.

SAUNA (HEAT HORMESIS)

Heat hormesis or sauna therapy is one of the most powerful medicines known to man. It is very well researched. One article showed massive reductions in cardiovascular disease and all-cause mortality in direct proportion to the frequency and length of time of sauna use. It is also very effective for chronic fatigue syndrome and for cutting pain and fatigue by more than half. Sauna also helped with brain fog, depression, and sleep.

COLD THERAPY

Cold temperature is another hormesis that stimulates your mitochondria. Cold thermogenesis is a form of cold therapy to create heat in your body. Examples are the Roman cold pools (frigidarium) or the Nordic swim in icy lakes. We can all do this by finishing a shower with thirty seconds of cold water (it's not so bad if you build up to it over several days).

When you lower your body temperature, your body will shiver to create heat. This burns fat and glycogen from your muscles. Once depleted of glycogen, you will produce testosterone and growth hormone. It reduces inflammation and insulin resistance, and stimulates autophagy and make new mitochondria. Cold exposure improves thyroid function and increased energy expenditure and fat loss. You don't need to be in icy water; cold water about 60 degrees F is adequate to stimulate your mitochondria. If you can find a lake or stream of this temperature, it is even better in nature. In the summertime, my favorite is Fallen Leaf Lake near Lake Tahoe.

Cold therapy can help tone your vagus nerve, the largest parasympathetic nerve that connects the brain stem with your heart, lungs, intestines, liver, spleen, and kidneys. A high vagal tone means you are can relax quickly after stress. This is important because you will have better blood sugar control and less chronic inflammation. Fat loss and better skin are added benefits. The key to thermogenesis is to start slow and build up resistance. Start by putting your face into ice water for five minutes for thirty days. Alternating warm and cold several times is also very beneficial hormesis for your mitochondria.

Cold therapy increases the amount of brown adipose tissue (BAT) in the body, which is particularly high in mitochondria, hence the color. It was once thought only newborns and children had it. Now we know white adipose tissue can undergo a process known as browning where it becomes like BAT with chronic cold exposure. Once activated, they increase the number of mitochondria by biogenesis.

Methods to achieve browning include repeated or chronic exposure to cold temperatures such as being in the cold during winter, turning down the thermostat at home in winter, and cold water therapy. BAT in adults improved insulin sensitivity and glucose metabolism. So you can save on your heating bill and become healthier at the same time!

Going from a hot sauna to cold shower or pool could increase BAT over time. The same goes for finishing a shower with a cold rinse of thirty seconds (probably easiest to do). BAT holds potential for treating obesity because they burn much more calories than white fat.

GROUNDING AND FOREST BATHING

To be grounded, literally, is to place our bare feet on the ground, whether it is soil, sand, grass or concrete, especially when they are moist or wet. The earth has a negative charge and our bodies are positive, so there is a better balance between the sympathetic and parasympathetic systems. It is believed that many modern chronic diseases are due to a lack of negative ions to counteract the positive charge of free radicals. We are always walking with rubber-soled shoes, which prevent the transfer of negative charge to our feet. They are some of the most powerful antioxidants and anti-inflammatories known to man.

The health benefits are numerous since they affect all body systems and cells, including mitochondria:

- Improves sleep quality and feeling of restfulness upon waking
- Reduces muscle stiffness and soreness

- Reduces chronic pain
- Normalizes the daily cortisol secretion pattern for more energy and sleep
- Reduces stress and stimulates the parasympathetic system and reduces the sympathetic system
- Reduces the severity of the inflammatory response after intense workouts
- Raises your heart rate variability (ability to respond to stimuli)
- Improves mood
- Thins your blood by increasing the negative charge on red blood cells (prevents clots)
- Increases EZ or structured water inside cells so they can hold a charge
- Increases tissue healing

Where should you ground? The best place is at the beach in or near the water barefoot (*no* sandals!). Next best is moist grass or dirt. Concrete and ceramic tiles are acceptable if not sealed or painted. Asphalt and wood are non-conductors. Unfortunately, this process is slow, so count on spending 80–120 minutes for the negative ions to get absorbed.

If you can't spend that much time outside, you can use a grounding pad under your feet or sheet on your bed. These need to be connected to the ground in your electrical outlet. They can be particularly beneficial if you live or work in a high rise since you hold more charge on your body, which has an increased health risk. Make sure you touch the grounding pad with bare feet. The easiest is to sleep on a grounded sheet, which is something I've done for several years. Exercising barefoot outdoors is also a wonderful routine to establish. You kill two birds with one stone!

Forest bathing—Shinren-yoku—is a common lifestyle habit for Japanese people It is a cornerstone of preventive health care and healing for them. Studies have shown it can boost immunity, energy, mood, relaxation, and sleep. Simply walk slowly (barefoot if you can) and be aware of the natural surroundings through all your senses and breathe in the air. You can also practice mindfulness (being in the present) or meditation while there. You develop a sense of connection to nature and each other through this experience.

LIGHT: GOOD AND BAD

Research shows that light is a nutrient that plays a critical function in signaling mitochondria. It can tell mitochondria what to do and when, and different color wavelengths send different messages. Light has been used as therapy in medicine for many years. This makes sense because the eyes contain one of the highest concentrations of mitochondria in the body and have a direct connection to the brain. So the eyes are extremely sensitive to light and may affect their energy production.

Our visual system requires up to 15% of our body's total energy output, mainly in visual processing in the brain. We spend more and more time on electronic screens, which require so much energy to process. If the mitochondrial energy output is low, you may suffer from brain fog, headaches, and visual perception of shades of gray. This can be used to diagnose your mitochondrial health. When your eyes have to function in unnatural spectrums of light, as in artificial light, it stresses your mitochondria, slows down energy production, and increases free radical damage. This may have serious consequence on your mental performance. Mitochondria communicate with each other, so stress to one organ can affect many other organs.

Today we are exposed to more unnatural light spectrums than ever before. Dave Asprey calls it "junk light" just like junk food because they both mess up our mitochondria. Our cells are programmed to respond to natural sunlight, which is a full-spectrum light. It has both visible wavelengths and invisible infrared, which is felt as heat. Artificial light has removed the infrared portion, which is necessary for living things including our mitochondria.

We now tend to avoid ultraviolet A and B light because of damage to the lens and fear of skin cancer (caused by ultraviolet light from the sun). We use sunglasses, tinted windows, and sunscreen to block them. Excessive UV light can damage our bodies but we require some to function. UVB is needed to activate vitamin D3 in the skin and to set our circadian rhythm.

Newer artificial lights like white LED and compact fluorescent light lack part of the sun's spectrum that our bodies need. They eliminate infrared (no heat), red and violet light, and amplify blue light. In the interest of saving electricity, we've created an inner energy crisis. These lights look really white but they emit five times the blue light than sunlight. Our mitochondria have to make a lot of extra energy to process the blue light and create free radicals in the process.

You feel the damage to the mitochondria as eyestrain, fatigue, and brain fog. Over time, this develops into age-related pathologies including cancer and macular degeneration (deterioration of the central area of the retina). This is already the leading cause of blindness in developed countries, affecting one-third of the population over seventy-five. As we use more junk light and electronic screens, this problem will escalate and start at much younger ages.

Natural sunlight also increases free radicals but they signal the production of more antioxidants. Blue light, however, causes an increase in free radicals but does not trigger the antioxidant production, so they cause cell damage. This damage is not limited to the eyes but also the skin, causing premature aging and wrinkling. So the more time you spend under junk light and screens, the more eye and brain damage and skin wrinkling.

Sunlight can also stimulate photosynthesis to take place in our cells similar to plants and bacteria. According to the Human Photosynthesis Study Group in Mexico, human retina, as well as every cell of our body, has the amazing capability of absorbing energy directly from water. Melanin, the dark pigment in our skin, hair, and retina, absorb sunlight and use it to split water atoms into hydrogen, oxygen, and four additional electrons. Dr. Arturo Herrera claims that hydrogen atoms are then sent to cells where it can be recombined with oxygen to produce energy to supplement glucose metabolism. Melanin acts like a catalyst which promotes the chemical reaction but is not consumed by it.

The Human Photosynthesis Study Center claims that one-third of the energy available to a human is produced by melanin absorbing sunlight to split water. One main source of energy of the body not derived from mitochondria is water. Normal cells possess the ability to communicate information within and between cells mediated through water molecules.

As we saw in the supplement section (nicotinamide riboside), artificial light causes a reduction of NAD^+ necessary to produce energy. This reduction can change the shape of the eyeball over time and you become nearsighted. Even in the short term, eyestrain makes your brain tired and can weaken your eyes.

Blue light at 480 nanometers activates special sensors in the eyes that prevent sleep by decreasing melatonin. It inhibits energy production (oxidative phosphorylation) thus leading to more free radicals that cause oxidative stress. This then causes inflammation in all parts of the body.

Artificial light at night will have a negative impact on the circadian rhythm. Sunlight exposure during the day produces serotonin, the feel-good neurotransmitter. This is converted to melatonin that helps you sleep. If you don't get exposed to sunlight during the day, you won't have enough melatonin to sleep well at night. You won't cycle through deep sleep for that brain "washing" to occur. Not unexpectedly, low melatonin is associated with cancer risk and weight gain because of its effect on sleep.

To block excessive LED or fluorescent light in the office and the computer, you can wear the orange glasses that block blue wavelength. You can do the same in the evening while watching TV or on the computer so you'll make more melatonin for sleep.

RED LIGHT THERAPY

In the natural world, there are two periods of red light, at sunrise, and before sunset. This sets our circadian rhythm and that of mitochondria. Today we spend little time outdoors in the sunshine. Most of our time is spent indoors under blue light staring at the computer screen with no trace of red, infrared or UV. No wonder our mitochondria are not performing well.

There are many health benefits to red light therapy. It penetrates deep through the skin (5–10mm) into muscle and joints. It is a powerful detoxifier to remove toxic mold and heavy metals like mercury and arsenic through sweat. Twenty to thirty minutes at 130 degrees can do wonders for joint or muscle pain. I say this from experience, as such exposure brought me relief when I had a severe pelvic muscle dysfunction. Each session should be followed by a cool to cold shower to close up the skin pores so that the toxins don't get reabsorbed back into the body. You will feel totally reinvigorated and re-energized.

Red and infrared light is well documented to make your mitochondria grow and produce more energy. It also stimulates collagen synthesis, which helps skin, connective tissue, bone, and joints. Collagen protein powder is very popular these days and I add it to my morning coffee followed by the sauna.

I also like the wearable wrap that has red and near-infrared LED lights that you can place on areas of pain, inflammation, or injury for quicker recovery. You can also wrap it around your head for the brain and to grow hair.

Red lasers can help people with Alzheimer's and other neurodegenerative diseases by decreasing amyloid plaques and increase BDNF and blood flow and decrease inflammation. For autism, a study showed impressive improvement compared to LED for home use.

STRUCTURED WATER AND HYDROGEN WATER

Dr. Gerald Pollack from the University of Washington discovered that the water in our cells is in a biologically active form called exclusion zone (EZ) or structured water or fourth phase water (in between solid and liquid). This water has a negative charge inside the cell and positive outside, so it acts as a battery and can store energy to distribute to areas of need. It is more viscous, dense, and alkaline than regular water. The best part is that it makes mitochondria stronger and produce more energy by transferring electrons down the ETC. EZ water is also an antioxidant and protects the cell from damage and cell aging. It can help proteins to fold properly by giving them energy. This allows for quicker recovery from stressors.

Besides red light, you can make EZ water by drinking fruit and vegetable juice, fresh spring water, and water agitated in a blender or vortex. The most natural way is exposure to sunlight on bare skin. Toxins from food and environment and junk light will decrease structured water. If you live in a place without much sun like the Pacific Northwest, use a UV sunlamp for ten minutes in the morning or a red LED light strip on your desk.

Hydrogen water is molecular hydrogen (H2) gas dissolved in water and is a powerful selective mitochondrial antioxidant and anti-inflammatory that has only gained interest since 2007 after an article was published in *Nature Medicine*.[14] Since then there have been more than a thousand scientific articles published demonstrating hydrogen's uses. It is the smallest molecule in the universe, is neutral and non-polar, and can easily penetrate any cell and organelle in the body. It is very stable and doesn't dissociate in water, so it will not alter the pH of water or our body. It has been found to be useful for a variety of conditions but mainly improves oxidative stress, which is the foundation of so many diseases. It selectively inhibits the most damaging free radicals, the hydroxyl and peroxynitrite radicals. It leaves alone the beneficial ones such as nitric oxide, which causes vasodilation in blood vessels and hydrogen peroxide, which kills microbes, or superoxide. Only hydrogen can bring a balance of oxidation and reduction to a cell. As a result, you see improvements in superoxide dismutase and glutathione levels, two useful antioxidants. It can also prevent free radicals from being produced in the first place.

Another mechanism of hydrogen is the activation of the Nrf2 pathway. This factor goes into the nucleus and binds to the DNA to activate the transcription of other cytoprotective enzymes such as glutathione, superoxide dismutase, catalase, etc.

Our intestinal microbiome ferment fiber and produce about two-and-a-half gallons of hydrogen gas per day, so we're always exposed to it. This indicates that there is complete safety for everybody regardless of dose. So why drink more in such low amounts? One study showed that intermittent exposure had the most effect. Apparently, continuous exposure leads to habituation.

Hydrogen therapy has been shown to be effective in several areas:
- Low blood flow causing stroke and heart attacks
- Neuroprotection in dementia, Parkinson's, depression
- Inflammation, wound healing, rheumatoid arthritis, colitis
- Metabolic syndrome: diabetes, arteriosclerosis, obesity
- Side effects of cancer therapies
- Mitochondrial diseases
- Anti-aging

Here are a few fascinating facts. Drinking hydrogen water had the same effect as restricting calories by about 20% similar to intermittent fasting. Another study showed molecular hydrogen effectively prevents liver damage (fatty liver) caused by a high sugar diet. It normalized impaired glucose tolerance in metabolic syndrome in a mechanism similar to insulin. There's also evidence that it can suppress cancer growth and lessen the toxicity of chemotherapy.

There are many ways to administer hydrogen. The easiest is dissolved in water to drink or bathe. You can inhale it through a nasal cannula or mask. It can be as an intravenous hydrogen saline injection or even hyperbaric hydrogen therapy. I personally have been using the Trusii tabletop machine that has the highest concentration of hydrogen water available on the market (around 9%). It also has an inhalation port with a nasal cannula. This machine has been very beneficial to me when I had severe hip and leg pain and stiffness after running an errand or a short workout at the gym. My pain was from a buildup of lactic acid from poor mitochondrial function. Hydrogen has been shown to reduce lactic acid in the body. I would come home and inhale hydrogen gas for about five minutes while drinking hydrogen water and can recover in that short amount of time.

The hydrogen level returns to baseline in about an hour but has residual therapeutic effects that last for days and even weeks. The reason is you're targeting gene expression, for example, the PGC-1 alpha gene, which is for mitochondrial biogenesis (the gene that I have a variant). By altering gene expression, some of the changes can last for some time. We end up with a greater density of mitochondria per cell in the needed areas.

MASSAGE AND BODY WORK

I'm sure you're familiar with massage as a way to relax tense muscles and feel good. A study from Canada shows that it can increase mitochondrial biogenesis and reduce inflammation. It increases blood flow to the massaged areas, which brings in more oxygen for aerobic respiration. It also drains the lymphatic fluid containing waste material from the tissue since there is no pump in the lymphatic system. Lymphatic massage should be in the direction of the heart where lymph is drained into the vein. Deep respiration and bouncing on a trampoline also helps drain lymphatics.

Deep tissue massage works on the muscles and fascia that cause chronic pain, posture, and mobility issues. It can rub out areas of tight muscles called knots that can improve posture and movement. It is also more condition-oriented than a relaxing massage, such as sports injuries, fibromyalgia, arthritis, repetitive strains, etc. This kind of massage helped my tight leg muscles. In a survey of 34,000 people in *Consumer Reports*, deep tissue massage was preferred over chiropractic, acupuncture, physical therapy, exercise, and medication. Removing the knots can definitely increase blood flow and bring oxygen to the muscles to boost mitochondrial function.

STEM CELLS THERAPY

Stem cells are undifferentiated cells that give rise to any type of cell in the body. They can come from our own body (somatic) or from an embryo. They are used to regenerate and repair diseased or damaged tissues. But as we age, their number decreases substantially from bone marrow and fat. Again, their functions are controlled by the health of your mitochondria. In other words, mitochondrial dysfunction will affect somatic stem cells and lead to tissue degeneration and premature aging. The accumulation of mtDNA mutations can disturb the redox homeostasis of stem cells and increase reactive oxygen species, rendering them less effective. Basically, mitochondrial integrity is essential for maintaining somatic stem cell homeostasis and the aging process. By keeping mitochondria healthy, we maintain the pool of stem cells that can regenerate new tissues and delay aging.

Stem cell therapy is a relatively new procedure where your own stem cells are collected from bone marrow or fat, get concentrated and activated and re-injected to the patient in areas of pain or injury.

PULSED ELECTROMAGNETIC FORCE (PEMF) THERAPY

PEMF therapy uses bursts of low-energy electromagnetic waves to heal damaged bone, soft tissues, injury, pain, and even stimulate internal organs. It passes through the skin and penetrates into deep tissue to activate natural cell repair. It can charge up your mitochondria directly, like plugging them into the socket. Perhaps the easiest way to understand PEMF is to think of each cell in your body as if it were a little battery. Like with any battery, sometimes your cells become tired and worn, whether due to age, stress, overuse, or damage, making it more difficult for them to fight off any type of potentially damaging force or illness.

Every disease in the body is preceded by a drop in the cell charge. Through PEMF therapy, your mitochondrial batteries essentially become recharged. The energy supplied via PEMF waves gives them the energy they need to ward off whatever is threatening them, whether it's a trauma or a disease-based threat. This makes it easier for the body to restore its health naturally, simply by using the electrical currents and impulses that are already interacting within and throughout their cells.

PEMF has been used to improve functions like:
- Immune function
- Sleep
- Soft tissue injury
- Bone fracture healing and density (osteoporosis)
- Depression and anxiety
- Blood circulation particularly microcirculation and viscosity
- Pain from chronic conditions and fibromyalgia
- Hormonal balance
- Regenerate nerves in the spinal cord and peripheral nerves
- Joint pain from osteoarthritis
- Diabetic ulcers
- Inflammatory skin conditions
- Liver detoxification
- Erectile dysfunction
- Burns

You may be concerned about EMF from cell phones, routers, microwaves, etc., damaging your DNA and causing cancer. They have a very high frequency, which can break off electrons from molecules and cause damage. PEMF's frequency is similar to what you find in nature, in the 5–30Hz range, which is less than what can be had from a thunderstorm. Furthermore, it is pulsed one to ten times per second and brief, lasting ten to twenty minutes per treatment. The rapid pulsing of EMF is much more effective than a non-pulsed one like a magnet since the body habituates to it. The treatment can be divided into several sessions in a day.

As we age, our circulation, particularly the microcirculation at the capillaries level, slows down and the red blood cells clump up. There is less delivery of oxygen and mitochondria are not able to make ATP. By boosting the microcirculation, red blood cells are free to flow and deliver their oxygen. You can see the change on microscopy after a single PEMF therapy. You need many treatments along with diet and lifestyle changes to maintain this change.

You can get PEMF mats to sleep on or lie on. Some of them are combined with near and far infrared lights, magnets, and stones like tourmaline, amethyst, and jade. They are generally under $1000 depending on the length.

EXTREME BIOHACKS

I just want to mention a few more extreme and expensive biohacks for those needing or wanting them or just to know about them. I have not personally tried them but Dave Asprey has felt benefits from them.

The first one is a hyperbaric oxygen therapy (HBOT) where the air is pressured with or without added oxygen. They are expensive to buy, but you can go to a center and pay by the session. The number of sessions depends on your condition. The conditions treated are ischemia (poor blood flow), gangrene, and non-healing wounds, in addition to decompression sickness and carbon monoxide poisoning.

Ozone therapy uses ozone, which is three oxygen atoms and gives it powerful healing properties. It regulates the immune system and fights infections and cancer. Ozone stimulates cells to take up more oxygen for the mitochondria and protect them against oxidative stress. The most powerful therapy is called major autohemotherapy (MAH) where blood is drawn, ozone gas is mixed into it and then gets reintroduced into your veins. You can also take ozone by insufflation vaginally or into the rectum. The third type is injecting ozone into an injury site or joint. Asprey says if you're dealing with early-onset mitochondrial dysfunction (EOMD), this therapy has the potential of prolonging their function for years. Shallenberger states in his book *The Ozone Miracle* that ozone stimulates the mitochondria ten times better than oxygen by using it more efficiently.

Cryotherapy is exposure to super-chilled air that is –270 F for up to three minutes. Again, Asprey claims there is no stronger mitochondrial recharge in that short time. It stimulates collagen synthesis in your skin, which means fewer wrinkles, especially with collagen protein.

A whole-body vibration platform is a device you stand on which vibrates thirty times per second compared to one bounce per second with a mini-trampoline. I have tried this and it's great for a quick break from sitting at the desk. It's like having a mini-workout without doing anything. These machines are pricey at over $1000. This speed of vibration will also accelerate the formation of structured water.

In the next chapter, we will examine the role of functional medicine in the diagnosis and treatment of mitochondrial dysfunction.

CHAPTER SUMMARY

1. Hormesis is any external stimulus that applied at a low level can stimulate mitochondria while it would have the opposite effect at a high level.
2. Biohacking is the art and science of exploiting hormesis to gain control over our own body.
3. Exercise, especially high-intensity interval training, is the most important hormesis for the mitochondria.
4. Optimize oxygen delivery to cells through proper breathing.
5. Optimize circadian rhythm (light and dark) and sleep.
6. Increase cell energetics with energy medicine: red light therapy, PEMF.

CHAPTER SIX

FUNCTIONAL MEDICINE APPROACH TO MITOCHONDRI-AL DYSFUNCTION

WHAT IS FUNCTIONAL MEDICINE?

Functional medicine is a branch of holistic or integrative medicine designed to examine the root cause of chronic diseases or conditions. It is functional systems-based rather than organ-based and is concerned with conditions versus diseases. These systems are detoxification, energy, defense, communication, structure, transport, and assimilation/elimination. Each system may involve several organs. The functional laboratory testing often looks deeper than the routine tests, even to the cellular level. The holistic aspect looks at the whole person body, mind, and spirit, and how imbalances in one affect the whole. In this respect, it is similar to Eastern or traditional medicine. Yet it is completely science-based in Western medicine.

The treatment is based on the fact the body can heal itself once we address the root imbalance(s). We try to avoid pharmaceutical medications with their side effects and prefer natural supplements, balanced diets, and healthy lifestyles. The supplements are used as a bridge while the diet and lifestyle habits are being established. It's like amending the soil so a beautiful garden can flourish and crowd out the weeds.

This treatment approach is shown to be increasingly the right one as we now know more about the microbiome in our gut. It is the central player in the genesis of diseases affecting many different organs that don't seem related. The microbiome is indeed like a garden of thousands of different species of bacteria, fungi, and viruses that all live in harmony and are very beneficial to health. However, once there is an overgrowth of one or more species, an imbalance exists and the beneficial ones may be diminished or lost. It's like an invasive plant starts to take over the garden and crowd out the more delicate plants. This is a condition called dysbiosis and is a major cause of leaky gut, immune dysfunction, and autoimmunity.

Functional medicine can also be characterized by the four Ps: personalized, proactive, predictive, and preventive. In other words, it is a treatment system personalized to your symptoms and root cause, genetics, environment, and lab findings. The patient needs to be proactively involved in his own care and healing process. The practitioner is like a coach to guide and oversee the process, but the work has to be done by the patient. The labs help to predict what systems are out of balance and where the patient is in the disease process. The whole goal is to prevent the late stage of disease when it is still easily reversible and before conventional medicine is needed.

Functional medicine is an integrative modality and welcomes all other forms of "alternative" therapies as long as they treat the whole patient and there are no significant side effects. Chiropractic care addresses the musculoskeletal system, which can have a major impact on overall health. Other modalities like traditional Chinese medicine, ayurvedic medicine, naturopathic medicine, acupuncture, herbalism, etc., can all help restore balance and allow the body to heal as a whole.

How are we able to find the root cause(s) when conventional doctors cannot? First, we use a detailed intake form that starts with prenatal history, followed by all possible antecedents (past contributors) that may have led up to the current complaints or condition. We also look for a trigger, usually a very stressful life event or illness, after which it has not been the same. Conditions that perpetuate the disease called mediators such as ongoing stress, hidden infection, sleep deprivation, etc., are examined. These conditions can be plotted on a timeline, which helps the patient see the history clearly. The diet, supplements, and medications are documented. This entire process may take more than an hour just to complete. It gives the practitioner a good handle on finding the root cause.

Second, the first appointment, usually one to one and a half hours, is just to go over the history and bring out significant history that the patient may not have remembered or connected. The appointment includes a physical exam to confirm or add to the pertinent history.

Third, functional lab testing is very different from conventional labs. They are not designed to diagnose a specific disease, but rather to find early signs of an impending disease process or trend while it's still reversible with natural therapies and lifestyle changes. We thus avoid the unnecessary use of drugs or surgery.

Oftentimes, even without getting to the deepest level of the root cause, functional medicine fixes the terrain of the body that's akin to improving the soil of a garden. It allows health to flourish, which naturally suppresses disease conditions similar to balancing the microbiome in the gut. The terrain would be like adequate sleep and rest, a balanced organic diet, hydration, and exercise.

My specific approach to functional medicine is based on that of my mentor Dr. Dan Kalish. He continues a long naturopathic tradition passed to him by his mentors. The Kalish method has been validated by the Mayo clinic in a study published in 2016 in *Complementary Therapies in Clinical Practice*.[15] Twenty-six middle-aged professional women complaining of stress, fatigue, digestive issues, and poor quality of life were treated for twenty-eight weeks. They were placed on an adrenal program, herbal treatment of H. pylori and parasites, and leaky gut protocol. They all had a salivary cortisol test, stool test, and organic acids test. The pilot study showed "significant improvements in many stress, fatigue, and quality of life measure." The Kalish method of treatment for these symptoms and conditions is the only one scientifically validated in functional medicine.

The Kalish method relies heavily on the state of the art functional laboratory testing. The tests were developed by

Dr. Richard Lord many years ago and he has been mentoring Dr. Kalish in recent years. I first learned about making a diagnosis of mitochondrial dysfunction from these mentors.

FUNCTIONAL LABORATORY DIAGNOSIS – THREE BODY SYSTEMS

In the Kalish method of functional medicine, we rely on three key tests: the organic acids test (urine), stool test, and salivary cortisol test.[16] These are required for all patients as they provide a complete picture of the three body systems: neuroendocrine system, GI system, and the detox system.

The neuroendocrine system includes adrenal and thyroid hormones, neurotransmitters, and energy production (mitochondrial function). The GI system includes pathogens, microbiome, leaky gut, and food sensitivities. The detox system reflects liver function, oxidative stress and methylation, and inflammation. These systems represent the order of disease formation starting with stress on the adrenal glands and leading to hormonal imbalances and an energy deficit. Over time, these imbalances lead to gut problems from erosion of the gut lining (catabolic state), dysbiosis and pathogens, and leaky gut. The latter leads to liver detoxification issues, inflammation, and oxidative stress. It is also a treatment map as a guideline to the order of treatment.

ORGANIC ACIDS TEST

One test that is done by all my patients regardless of symptoms is the organic acids test originally developed by Dr. Lord.[17] This test looks at forty-six markers of energy metabolism, liver detoxification, brain neurotransmitters, and gut health. Energy metabolism is separated into fatty acid metabolism, carbohydrate metabolism, Krebs cycle (citric acid cycle) energy production, and protein metabolism (also B vitamin markers). These four groups constitute the first twenty-one markers. According to Dr. Lord, if six or more markers are low out of the first twenty-one, this indicated mitochondria failure.

We then need to go upstream to each food component: carbohydrates, fat, and protein to see if it is properly metabolized into the right molecule that can then feed into the Krebs cycle and the ETC to produce energy. If you're not able to burn fat into energy, then carnitine will enhance this step. If there's a blockage in the metabolism of carbohydrates, chromium and lipoic acid can jump-start this step. The metabolism of amino acids needs various B vitamins, which should be replaced if insufficient. The Krebs cycle itself may have certain steps that are slowed due to lack of micronutrients and B vitamins. Again, they need to be replaced along with CoQ-10. There are combination products that contain all the necessary ingredients for mitochondrial support.

Another category of markers is known as methylation cofactors, which also reflect mitochondrial function. In short, methylation is a biochemical process of transferring a methyl group to another substance. This process is needed for hundreds of critical chemical reactions throughout the body such as DNA regulation and energy metabolism. Sixty percent of people have a genetic mutation that depletes the body of methylation, and the diet is often inadequate. They require supplementation with vitamin B-9 as methylfolate.

One section of the organic acids test is devoted to liver detoxification, both phase 1 and 2 as well as glutathione level. Products are available to support all three areas.

The neurotransmitter section is another critical part of the test. It looks at the urinary metabolites of catecholamines, dopamine, and serotonin. These are the major neurotransmitters that determine mood: anxiety, depression, and lack of motivation. Markers of brain inflammation are also in this section. You then have to look into the cause of the inflammation, most likely from the gut via the gut-brain connection.

The final section of the organic acids test is gut microbiome including fungi. The bacterial metabolism can indirectly show the presence of dysbiosis (imbalance). It can also show the polyphenol consumption in your diet. Last but not least, there is a marker for yeast overgrowth that needs to be addressed with diet.

As you can see, this test constitutes the most important survey of the main body systems. It provides concrete clues to the underlying cause(s) and directs the practitioner to the treatment plan.

STOOL TEST

The second critical test that I have all my patients take is a stool test. The first section looks for bacterial, viral, and parasitic pathogens (capable of causing illness). It then looks for the presence of Helicobacter pylori, the bacteria that causes gastric ulcers. Another section identifies the opportunistic bacteria (can be harmful if in excess) that can trigger autoimmune diseases or dysbiosis. Similarly, there's a section identifying the parasites that may be opportunistic given the right environment. Several main yeasts and fungi are examined as well.

The final section of the test looks at digestive enzymes and the amount of fat in the stool. The gut immune response known as secretory IgA shows if there's a reaction to infection or the gluten molecule gliadin. These are clues to the presence of food sensitivities and activation or depression of gut immunity. The zonulin marker indicates the presence of leaky gut syndrome.

This test must be done whether or not the patient has gut symptoms. Too many times there are hidden pathogens and parasites that have been present for many years and the symptoms are either ignored or very low grade. A bad diet can exacerbate the bacterial imbalance and overgrowth of yeasts.

The consequences of dysbiosis, we now know, are catastrophic and the root cause of most of the major degenerative diseases throughout the body. Pathogenic overgrowth causes the single-cell lining on the inside of the small bowel to become "leaky" so that partially digested food particles and pathogens can now pass into the blood stream and cause a major immune response. Seventy to eighty percent of our immune cells are located under the intestinal cell lining and react to pathogens and unrecognized food particles. Over time and with each meal the gut becomes more and more inflamed. The immune system becomes dysregulated and starts to attack our own tissue because of the molecules resembling food particles that leak through. You now have developed autoimmunity. If it attacks the thyroid, you have Hashimoto's thyroiditis. If it attacks joints, you have rheumatoid arthritis. If it attacks the brain, you get cerebellar ataxia. If it attacks blood vessels, you get lupus.

Altogether there are now over one hundred disease conditions under the umbrella of autoimmune diseases. These disorders have been rising exponentially in the last twenty years. There is generally a genetic predisposition underlying autoimmunity. The specific tissue under attack is wherever the weakest link in the chain is. Fatigue is often associated with these conditions because of the damage to mitochondria from inflammation.

SALIVARY CORTISOL TEST

The third lab test in the Kalish method is the salivary cortisol test. Cortisol is the main hormone produced by the adrenal glands, which sit on top of the kidneys. Cortisol is the body's stress hormone that is secreted in a predictable diurnal pattern. It is highest after awakening in the morning, then falls through the day and is lowest at night before bedtime. The test also measures DHEA, a hormone that is a precursor to the sex hormones estrogen and testosterone.

Under normal circumstances, cortisol is elevated in acute situations by a stressor such as running to catch a bus and drops down when you're on the bus. But in the modern era when stress is constant and unrelenting, the rhythm regulated by the brain known as the HPA axis becomes abnormal. Over time, the body's production of cortisol comes at the expense of progesterone and DHEA and sex hormones (cortisol steal). This means that under constant stressful situations, the body shifts away from reproduction to deal with stress. Cortisol also harms the brain and cause brain fog and poor memory.

Stress is not just emotional but can also come from bad diet, pain, and inflammation. Emotional stress from the death of loved ones and divorce is always the most significant even if several years have passed. Dietary stress results from poor blood sugar control from too much sugar and carbohydrates. Insulin and cortisol fight to control the sugar and both end up adding fat to the abdomen. Unless the blood sugar and cortisol are stabilized, it is very hard to lose belly fat.

The third form of stress is from pain and inflammation. Inflammation in the gut can be from food sensitivities such as gluten or from hidden pathogens and parasites. High cortisol is initially anti-inflammatory but prolonged elevation suppresses the immune system. You become very susceptible to colds and flu and other infections.

Stage one of adrenal fatigue shows very high cortisol levels throughout the day and high DHEA. A typical patient is on the go day and night, skips meals, has late afternoon crash, craves caffeine in morning and sugar in afternoon, and feels wired and tired. She might only get a couple of hours of sleep at night after taking care of the kids.

After several years of stage one, you progress to stage two with low to normal total cortisol and lower DHEA. Symptoms like fatigue, weight gain, depression, non-restorative sleep, and digestive disorders appear.

Stage three is adrenal exhaustion with very low total cortisol and DHEA. These might be the successful business owners who feel responsible for the whole company and family too. Exercise becomes impossible. He can barely get through the day. Depression sets in more along with aches and pain all over.

Functional medicine can really shine in this condition, as it can reverse the adrenal changes in a matter of months. We use low-dose pregnenolone and DHEA, precursors to cortisol and sex hormones. We raise cortisol with licorice and lower it by phosphorylated serine. Blood sugar support with lipoic acid and adaptogenic herbs like ashwagandha are also used along with high dose vitamin C. The goal is to re-establish the brain-adrenal connection to the normal circadian pattern.

These supplements are the temporary bridge to establishing a proper diet, exercise and lifestyle changes. Once the patient can see the disruption in their rhythm, they become motivated to make changes. The diet should avoid sugar and excessive carbohydrates so that the blood glucose remains more stable and there are no swings in insulin or cortisol reactions. The blood sugar is usually a factor when daytime cortisol is out of balance. I recommend going gluten- and dairy-free.

The type and time of exercise can also be tailored to the cortisol pattern. During high cortisol, yoga, tai chi, or qigong may be a more appropriate exercise to do. Aerobic exercises may be more beneficial for low-cortisol times. Hard and prolonged aerobic exercise is not recommended for those with adrenal burnout.

Meditation practices can be very beneficial to anyone with high cortisol levels. The benefits of meditation have been well studied. There is a decrease in the cortisol levels after meditation. The meditation sessions can be timed with periods of high cortisol to bring it down. This is critical if one has high levels at night, because it's associated with obsessive worrying and inability to sleep.

If you have trouble waking up in the morning and the cortisol is low, you need bright, full-spectrum light (not fluorescent) to hit your eyes and release cortisol. Don't stay in bed in the dark and check emails. It's best to go outdoors and do light exercises and deep breathing. This is really important if you have an autoimmune disease because cortisol suppresses the T immune cells responsible for the symptoms. Light upon awakening will prevent the development of autoimmunity. Coffee can also help raise cortisol.

People with abnormal brain-adrenal rhythm need to follow a strict circadian rhythm. They need to rise, sleep, and eat at the same time and follow routines. Restful and deep sleep is mandatory to heal adrenal fatigue. Spend time in natural sunlight during the day and avoid fluorescent light. In the evening, use blue light blockers because that wavelength inhibits melatonin necessary for sleep. Avoid the use of screens one hour before bed.

TREATMENT OF MITOCHONDRIAL DYSFUNCTION

Once we make the diagnosis of mitochondrial dysfunction, what can we do to hopefully reverse it in time before there is significant symptoms or organ failure? Treatment of mitochondrial failure needs to be started early in the overall treatment plan. Without cellular energy, treatment of other body systems often fails. For example, treating low thyroid hormone with low or non-functional mitochondria is like turning up the thermostat without electricity or gas in the furnace. Detoxification by the liver will not work without energy too. The adrenal protocol will also not be effective.

The treatment in this situation involves high doses of free-form amino acids powder taken as a bolus. Additional tryptophan is added, as it's a rate-limiting (slowest) step in the synthesis of proteins. CoQ10 and magnesium, as well as a mitochondrial support formula, are also needed. Recently a product known as PQQ has become popular to enhance new mitochondria formation and function. This protocol needs to be used daily for at least two months depending on the severity and duration of the failure. Within a few weeks, a patient will begin to feel less fatigued and depressed and may even start to lose some weight. The development of full-blown chronic diseases has been averted.

If intervention is not undertaken at this early stage, continued oxidative stress will result in end-organ damage as diagnosed in conventional medicine. The following diseases have been associated with mitochondrial damage: neurodegenerative brain diseases like Parkinson's and Alzheimer's, immune system disorders, cardiovascular and hepatic diseases. This makes sense since these organs have lots of mitochondria and use a high percentage of the body's energy. The brain and nervous system use 25%–30% of the body's total energy. The heart is always beating thus requiring energy. The immune system when fighting infections is a major consumer. The liver needs energy to perform its digestive, metabolic, and detoxification functions. Obviously, when energy can't meet the demand, there is less-than-optimal function and the patient becomes symptomatic and performance suffers. The symptoms may be cognitive impairment, nerve pain, high blood sugar, chronic fatigue syndrome, or multiple chemical sensitivities.

When this process becomes chronic, the mitochondria involutes and the inner membrane folds break down. This triggers apoptosis, which is more beneficial than a necrotic death where the cell bursts open and the contents contaminate the surrounding cells and cause a chain reaction leading to extensive dead tissue zones.

GENERAL FUNCTIONAL MEDICINE APPROACH TO PATIENT WORKUP

Let's see how we can apply the Kalish method to typical patients that come to my office. You will see how all our body systems are interconnected. In the functional medicine way of thinking, everything can cause and be caused by everything else. The sequence of treatment is also critical, as the healing of one system affects that which is downstream. You will see how treatment is in the order of formation of the imbalances. For example, stress is usually the antecedent and trigger, which then sets off a predictable sequence or cascade of body system dysfunction. The number and severity of dysfunction are often dependent on the length of time and magnitude of the stress.

The mental, dietary, and inflammatory stressors result in adrenal fatigue followed by exhaustion. This process no doubt parallels mitochondrial dysfunction and poor energy production. The adrenal degeneration triggers gut problems due to the breakdown of the gut lining for energy, which then causes leaky gut, inflammation and subsequent food sensitivities and gut infections and dysbiosis. Gut inflammation then puts a burden on the liver detoxification system and block the absorption of nutrients in the gut, causing nutritional deficiencies. Gut inflammation also causes brain inflammation and neurotransmitter malfunction and mood disorders.

The sequence of treatment starts with the first system impacted by stress: the endocrine system with adrenals, thyroid, and sex hormones. The adrenal protocol is key to this part of the treatment. The patient will start to feel better fairly quickly. If there is mitochondrial failure, I like to give mitochondrial support at this early phase in order to have energy to heal each system.

The next phase involves the GI system, which comprises four components: pathogens, digestion, leaky gut, and microbiome/dysbiosis. The adrenal program would have improved the gut lining already. The killing of pathogens takes center stage here and usually involves a combination of herbal products and probiotics. Digestion is supported by enzymes and leaky gut with bone broth and L-glutamine. The gut program will be for two to four months depending on how many supplements the patient is willing to take at any one time.

Once the gut is treated we can now move to the detoxification phase. This phase may involve oxidative stress reduction and methylation support. Nutrient replacement may be done in this phase too. The preparation for detoxification is opening all means of drainage of lymph, bile, stool, sweat, and urine. Once these are flowing freely, the critical liver detoxification can begin.

Liver detoxification is divided into two phases. Phase I, known as Cytochrome P-450 enzymes, converts a lipid-soluble toxin to a more water-soluble intermediate metabolite. The biochemical reactions here include oxidation, reduction, hydrolysis, and dehalogenation. The nutrients used are B vitamins, glutathione, branched-chain amino acids, flavonoids, and phospholipids. Many harmful reactive oxygen intermediates are produced that can cause secondary tissue damage. Antioxidant-protective nutrients are needed here, particularly CoQ-10, silymarin (milk thistle), and vitamins A, C, and E.

Phase II, known as conjugation pathways, take the intermediary metabolites from phase I and turn them into polar water-soluble substances that can be excreted in bile, stool, and urine. The biochemical reactions here are sulfation, glucuronidation, glutathione conjugation, methylation, and amino acid conjugation. The nutrients used are sulfur-containing amino acids glycine, glutamine, cysteine, N-acetyl-cysteine, and methionine.

The treatment supports both phases of liver detoxification but particularly phase II. There are supplements that are a mixture of ingredients that help each phase. Glutathione is the main detox antioxidant molecule found in every cell of the body. It has many important functions including DNA synthesis and immune function. Glutathione also breaks down free radicals, regenerates vitamins C and E, and transports mercury out of the brain. Details of this product are in Chapter Four.

GUT HEALTH AND MITOCHONDRIA

We now know our microbiome in the gut controls so many of our body functions, from digestion, immune function, to brain function and mood. The microbiome is the entire community of bacteria, fungi, and viruses that co-exist in the gut. It feeds off the food we consume and in return, provide many benefits to us such as make vitamins and neurotransmitters. They outnumber human cells by a factor of ten and their genome by a factor of one hundred. Frequently today, it is out of balance, what we call dysbiosis, and certain species show an overgrowth, which may be pathogenic. Other times there may be a lack of certain species that are needed for gut health. This microbiome certainly affects our mitochondria and vice-versa since they can communicate with each other (they are both bacteria). We also know the microbiome changes in old age along with a weakened immune system, indicating they develop and age together.

Aging research has experienced tremendous progress with the idea that aging could be influenced by maintaining a healthy microbiome and gut function.[18] Exposure to multiple drugs and antibiotics, diet changes from poor digestion and absorption, increased permeability and inflammation and constipation all accompany aging and affect the microbiome. In short, maintaining gut and microbiome health has become another area of biohacking to delay the aging process.

It is found that older people have a different microbiome compared to healthy adults, which may be attributed to changes in lifestyle and diet. They have less microbial diversity, fewer commensals (non-pathogenic), and more opportunists (potentially causing harm) such as C. difficile. They also have lower short-chain fatty acids (SCFA), which are critical for gut health. So a restoration to a younger adult microbiome may prolong longevity.

Since gut health is my area of expertise and the foundation of functional medicine, maintaining a balanced microbiome needs to be a very important lifestyle factor. We know the gut is the starting point of all chronic diseases including autoimmune, neurodegenerative, and cardiovascular, which all involve inflammation. We also know inflammation can switch off mitochondrial energy production into cell defense and lowers the resilience threshold, making us susceptible to age-related disease. Therefore, keeping the gut and related organs such as liver and pancreas in optimal condition should be a pillar of lifestyle, dietary, and supplement regimen. It's also important to keep in mind that digestion and absorption are highly energy-dependent, so we need those mitochondria to work at full capacity.

Digestion starts with the right attitude of gratitude and rest, not an interruption to our work. This stimulates the parasympathetic system that increases the digestive enzymes and motility of the gut. Next, we have to chew the food at least twenty to thirty times until it is like pulp and allow time for the salivary enzyme to break down carbohydrates. It's also important not to drink beverages just before or during the meal because doing so dilutes the gastric acid and makes the stomach less acidic. This is critical for breakdown of proteins which otherwise could cause fermentation in the gut. The gallbladder needs to function properly for the bile to emulsify fat. The pancreas needs to secrete its enzymes that further break down food. Another part of the pancreas secretes insulin to bring down the blood sugar. We need to eat food with a low glycemic index so we don't overtax its secretion leading to insulin resistance.

In the small intestines, absorption of nutrients takes place through tiny finger-like projections called villi that increase the surface area to that of a tennis court. With exposure to medications and food sensitivities as well as toxins and pathogens, the surface lining cells become permeable which causes inflammation and blunting in the villi. Nutrient deficiencies may develop from improper absorption. There may be small intestinal bacterial overgrowth (SIBO) or fungal overgrowth (SIFO).

In the colon, the microbiome's number of different species (diversity), number of organisms, and the right ratio of phyla are all important. Pathogens need to be treated so that the microbiome may rebalance. All this information can be obtained with a functional stool test, especially using DNA testing of the organisms. This test should be done annually or if there is a change in bowel habits such as after a foreign trip.

The effect of food on the microbiome is critical to maintaining balance (homeostasis). Prebiotics provide fiber to feed good bacteria in the colon. The role of probiotics is both direct by changing the microbiome while passing through but not colonizing, and indirect by changing the immune system. If your diet is less than optimal, it is best to supplement with probiotics, especially if you have digestive symptoms. Better yet, eat homemade yogurt and other fermented foods like kimchi, kefir, sauerkraut, and tempeh. Your diet should also have abundant polyphenols from vegetables and fruits that also feed the beneficial microbiome since they are large molecules that can't be absorbed in the gut. There are now specialized microbiome stool tests that tell you what you should eat or not eat (Viome, a personalized health and wellness app, is one resource).

For those with low gastric acid secretion, use betaine hydrochloride to increase absorption of calcium, iron, and vitamin B-12. If pancreatic enzymes are low, take digestive enzymes that breakdown fat, protein, and carbohydrates. For slow bile flow, take phosphatidylcholine as supplement or eggs and cruciferous vegetables.

To have a healthy microbiome, it's important to avoid antibiotics, alcohol, antacids, and proton pump inhibitors, steroids, etc. A single course of antibiotics can alter the microbiome for many months. If you have to use it, take a probiotic in between the antibiotics. Eating a wide variety of fruits and vegetables with colors of the rainbow is always beneficial for the diversity of the microbiome.

CASE STUDIES

The five top symptoms readily treated with functional medicine are stress and fatigue, weight gain, anxiety/depression, digestive issues, and hormonal imbalance. Let's look at how we would approach them at my clinic through case studies without using pharmaceutical drugs. Remember, the earlier you start to tackle these issues, the easier they are reversed.

Mary, age fifty-five, came to see me for increasing job stress and fatigue, anxiety and depression, twenty-five pounds overweight, and unable to shed a pound no matter how she dieted. She's a successful executive with a ten-hour workday, with a husband and two teenagers at home. Her diet is standard American and getting worse with more sugar cravings most of the time and coffee during work and many skipped meals. On top of that, she has to travel out of town every other week for 2–3 days. This means frequent disruption of her circadian rhythm and it takes her longer to recover. She seems to catch a cold or flu after many trips, which further delays the recovery. This had been going on for about three years when her husband wanted a divorce and left with the boys. All of a sudden she's now alone at night and she started drinking one, then two glasses of wine and frequently a whole bottle in the evenings. She is even less inclined to cook and most dinners are eating out or take-outs. She now has very disrupted sleep, falling asleep easily after the wine, then waking up at 2 a.m. and unable to fall asleep until 4 a.m. She wakes to her alarm clock at 6:30 very groggy until she can have her first of several strong cups of coffee. After her coffees, she gets nauseated and more frequent bloating after meals. Her primary care doctor prescribed an anti-depressant, antacids, a proton pump inhibitor, and sleeping pills, which made her even groggier in the morning. She knew this was not the answer to her problems. Luckily, a work associate recommended functional medicine. When she came to see me, she was at the end of her rope.

She willingly did the saliva cortisol test, stool test, and organic acids test. The cortisol test showed a stage three adrenal fatigue with low total cortisol and DHEA, and the pattern shows very low morning, high noon, and low afternoon. This yoyo effect is very symptomatic for the patient alternating between tired and wired. She's placed on a stage three protocol with pregnenolone and DHEA and licorice for the low points and phosphatidyl serine for the peaks. General adrenal support with adaptogens, vitamin C, and lipoic acid for blood sugar support were also prescribed for two months. Her energy and mood swings improved within several weeks.

The stool test revealed Helicobacter pylori and Blastocystic hominis as two main pathogens that need to be eliminated. The first organism can cause gastric ulcers and reflux. The second one is a single-celled parasite that may or may not be symptomatic. There was also overgrowth of bacterial flora consistent with dysbiosis. She also had yeast overgrowth and leaky gut from the infections and dysbiosis. The herbal products for the killing phase followed the adrenal treatment along with probiotics for two months. Her reflux and bloating improved. A ketogenic diet was instituted with the elimination of dairy, sugar, and alcohol. Her weight finally began to come down and at the end of this three-month treatment phase, she had lost ten pounds and she felt great. She even began to take a walk after dinner instead of a second or third glass of wine.

The organic acids test showed ten of the first twenty-one metabolic markers low consistent with mitochondrial failure. She had trouble metabolizing fat, carbs, proteins, and in the Kreb cycle intermediates. No wonder she can't lose weight—she was lacking the enzyme carnitine to burn the fat for energy. She lost another ten pounds on carnitine and mitochondria support.

The neurotransmitter markers showed high catecholamines, low dopamine, and high normal serotonin, which is artificially inflated by her SSRI anti-depressant (would have been low without it). This accounts for her work stress, fatigue, and anxiety/depression. Simple amino acids tyrosine and 5-HTP in the right ratio was enough to improve her mood and wean off her medication.

This test also showed liver detoxification problems with low glutathione, which is due to the leaky gut and inflammation. You can treat this with liposomal glutathione for better absorption or N-acetylcholine, which is the precursor form. She was able to tolerate the mitochondria support, the neurotransmitter treatment, and the liver detoxification support all together following the gut treatment.

To review, on a cellular level, Mary's mitochondrial function has been seriously compromised from emotional, dietary, and inflammatory stress. The stress took a toll on her gut health and brain function as well as liver detoxification. By treating in phases starting with the oldest antecedents and triggers, the problems are eliminated one by one as the dead mitochondria are removed and new ones are made. This gives the cell the energy it needs to function properly.

Another case study is Janet, a forty-three-year-old home-maker who has a family history of autoimmune diseases and has had irritable bowel syndrome (IBS) with constipation since high school. Her diet was standard American with lots of sweets and fried foods and no vegetables other than potatoes. She had bad acne in school and later on, she was diagnosed with psoriasis. She became depressed and socially isolated. At the age of twenty-seven, her mother passed away from breast cancer and triggered massive panic attacks. After her first baby was born, she had severe postpartum depression and Hashimoto's thyroiditis. Five years later she developed intense joint pain and inflammation diagnosed as rheumatoid arthritis. By the time she came to see me, she looked twenty years older and had all the top five symptoms of Hashimoto's thyroiditis: fatigue, obesity, depression, gut problems, and female hormone imbalance (premature peri-menopause).

The triad of lab tests showed adrenal exhaustion stage 3, as expected. The gut pathogens cryptosporidium and giardia were found, as well as Klebsiella pneumoniae and Proteus mirabilis, which are associated with autoimmune triggers.

Yeasts Candida species and Geotrichum species were present. Gut inflammation marker and immune response to gluten were very elevated. Organic acids test showed mitochondria failure, low methylation, low neurotransmitters, and detoxification problem.

The treatment sequence follows the sequence of causation of the imbalances. We started with adrenals along with diet and lifestyle changes: no gluten, dairy, and sugar, no drugs or alcohol, and a routine of sleep, wake, and meals. Low dose pregnenolone and DHEA were given to reset the HPA axis along with adaptogens, vitamin C and multivitamins. This continued for six months before the cortisol curve started to normalize.

The next phase of treatment was to kill the gut pathogens using a combination of herbs for two months. This was followed by restoration of gut enzymes and stomach acid and healing the intestinal lining with glutamine and bone broth.

The final phase was to restore the mitochondrial function with free form amino acids, CoQ10, PQQ, magnesium, and oxygen through deep breathing exercises. This was followed by liver detox support, methylation support with B12 and methylfolate, and neurotransmitter rebalancing for a better mood.

AUTOIMMUNE DISEASES

I like to discuss Janet's case as an illustration of autoimmune diseases, a condition I treat frequently. There are three factors necessary for its formation: genetic predisposition (family history), leaky gut, and immune dysregulation. The genetics might determine what organ(s) might be affected, the so-called weak link in the chain. Leaky gut can be from a host of causes, from pathogens, dysbiosis from bad diet, medications, or stress. The leaky lining allows undigested food particles to enter the blood stream where it is seen as foreign and causes an inflammatory response in the form of antibodies. There is often molecular mimicry (similarity) between the protein food particles and the protein in our organs such as the thyroid. These antibodies will start to damage the tissue and cause symptoms and eventually full-blown disease after many years. The immune system loses its ability to tell between self and non-self (immune tolerance). We now know that the antibodies can be present for years before symptoms in a subclinical stage, and if treatment is started at this point, we can prevent the disease. You know something is wrong at this stage but your doctor tells you everything's fine or gives you an anti-depressant.

There are now more than 120 autoimmune diseases. It is one of the fastest-growing diseases in the last twenty years affecting fifty to seventy million Americans. It ranks number three in sickness and deaths behind cardiovascular disease and cancer. It is also very expensive to treat using conventional drugs like Humira costing $5500 per injection.

Autoimmunity can affect many different organs and tissues. Some of the most common ones are Hashimoto's and Grave's disease in the thyroid, lupus in blood vessels, rheumatoid arthritis in joints, multiple sclerosis in the brain, and inflammatory bowel disease and celiac disease in the gut. Functional medicine is the most effective way to stop and reverse the process by treating the underlying causes. Most if not all autoimmune diseases involve mitochondrial dysfunction, which is the cause of fatigue. Applying the Kalish method, I would do the three tests and treat adrenal fatigue, gut issues, and mitochondrial energy production.

In the next chapter, we will examine in depth the main mitochondria-related diseases. You may be surprised that they are the main chronic diseases that plague our country today.

CHAPTER SUMMARY

1. Functional medicine is a holistic and integrative medicine that looks for root causes of a series of seemingly unrelated symptoms and is treated with diet, supplements, and lifestyle changes.
2. Functional medicine uses functional lab testing to find the root causes. These include salivary cortisol, stool, and organic acids test.
3. Mitochondrial dysfunction is diagnosed by the organic acids test.
4. Mitochondrial dysfunction is treated with free-form amino acids, CoQ10, magnesium, and oxygen (proper breathing).
5. The functional medicine paradigm is that all diseases start with stress and gut imbalance producing liver detoxification deficiency and accumulation of toxic load, oxidative stress, and loss of mitochondrial function.

6. Chronic autoimmune diseases are increasing exponentially today and functional medicine is best equipped to control or reverse it.

CHAPTER SEVEN

MITOCHONDRIAL DISEASES

There are two sets of genomes involved in making mitochondria work, mtDNA (maternal) and nDNA (both parents), so inheritance patterns can range greatly. There are countless interactions between them. The variation in mtDNA in the mother's eggs is surprisingly high. The onset of symptoms in this group of diseases can vary by decades, and even between siblings with the identical genetic mitochondrial mutation.

Currently, there are over two hundred known types of mitochondrial mutations, and a wide range of common degenerative diseases have been found to involve one or more of these mutations. These mutations cause the mitochondria to stop making energy, which leads to cell death. When the energy requirements can no longer be fully met, the symptom manifests as fatigue. They mainly affect the brain, nerves, muscles, heart, kidneys, and glands: all organs with a high demand for energy. For a particular tissue or organ to become dysfunctional, a critical number of its mtDNA must be defective, called the threshold effect. Each organ has a different threshold, energy requirement, and sensitivity to free radical damage. All these factors combine to determine how it will respond to genetic damage.

When a cell divides, its mitochondria are distributed at random between the two daughter cells. One might inherit all the defective mitochondria, the other all healthy ones. The cell with all defective mitochondria will die by apoptosis. Each cell has different mitochondria with different mtDNA known as heteroplasmy. The degree of heteroplasmy also differs from organ to organ and cell to cell, leading to a vast range of possible disease symptoms. A genetic defect may be prominent if it occurs in a fast-replicating cell or minor if in a slow-replicating one. All these factors make it almost impossible to predict how the disease will progress in any one individual. Even many common degenerative diseases such as cardiovascular diseases, cancers, and dementia are now seen as specific mitochondrial diseases.

SYMPTOMS OF MITOCHONDRIAL DYSFUNCTION

In the early stage of dysfunction, the symptoms are non-specific. There might be disruption of your normal sleep pattern, like becoming a night owl if you normally sleep at 10 p.m. You need caffeine and sugar to get through the slumps in your day. There might be easy fatigue and less endurance in normal activities or exercise. You could have mood swings, anxiety, and depression for no reason. You could also have vague muscle and joint pain all over the body. You may experience mental fog and decreased memory.

In the late stage, you feel severe fatigue, pain, and slow recovery from slight exertion or exercise. The mental fog and memory loss become more profound. There is now dizziness, severe anxiety and depression, cardiac problems, and shortness of breath. The body becomes more acidic from a build-up of lactic acid in the muscles from anaerobic respiration. This can manifest as fibromyalgia.

The goal is to maximize the delivery of energy by mitochondria and minimize the wasted expenditure of energy in the form of emotional stress, infections, inflammation, and autoimmunity.

DIABETES, TYPE 2

Diabetes and insulin resistance is a major and growing medical problem today. New research points to the mitochondria as the culprit. As we age, our mitochondria deteriorate and there's a decline in the rate of fat oxidation and production of energy. This predisposes us to fat accumulation in muscle and liver. The mitochondria in the beta cells that make insulin in the pancreas slow down resulting in impaired glucose tolerance, hyperglycemia, and eventually type 2 diabetes. High blood sugar induces mitochondrial superoxide production in the endothelial cells, which are an important mediator of diabetic complications such as atherosclerosis, hypertension, heart failure, and premature aging. It also will react with proteins to form advanced glycation end products (AGEs), which can also bind to mitochondria and compromise their function.

The mitochondria are smaller than normal and accumulate lipids because they can't metabolize fatty acids for energy in the Krebs cycle. PGC-1alpha, an enzyme located in the mitochondrial matrix for lipid metabolism, is found to be reduced in type 2 diabetes. The accumulated lipids turn into cytotoxic compounds called lipid peroxides (lipotoxicity), thereby further damaging the mitochondria, thus leading to insulin resistance.

The chain of events is as follows:
1. Mitochondrial damage in the target cells such as muscles results in lipid peroxide accumulation.
2. Lipid peroxide accumulation results in insulin resistance.
3. Beta cells in the pancreas must increase their metabolism to create more insulin which requires more energy.
4. Over time, the beta cells accumulate damage to their mitochondria due to high metabolism and energy demand.
5. Beta cells start to die off, resulting in a drop in insulin and elevated blood glucose as seen in uncontrolled type 2 diabetes.

There is also a rare form of mitochondrial diabetes presenting in middle age, which starts as a mtDNA defect, so it is maternally transmitted, and associated with hearing loss. There is decreased insulin secretion but not insulin resistance, suggesting the problem is in the mitochondria of beta cells. The mutation leads to defects in mitochondrial proteins, ending in mitochondrial dysfunction.

This spiraling process can be stopped and even reversed by a combination of calorie restriction and exercise. A study found that middle-aged obese diabetics who reduced calorie intake by 25% and engaged in moderate exercise for four months boosted their mitochondria density by 67%!

Another study in 2011 showed a severely calorie-restricted diet of only 600 calories per day for eight weeks reversed diabetes in 100% of participants. What was once thought to be a lifelong, irreversible condition can be reversed and they remained diabetes-free as long as they maintained the calorie restriction. The pancreas was found to regain its production of insulin, and muscles and liver became sensitive to insulin again. This was confirmed by a study from Canada in 2017. We might need to reclassify diabetes as a metabolic disease rather than endocrine because it's not insulin resistance that's the root of the problem, but poor mitochondrial function.

CARDIOVASCULAR DISEASE

Cardiovascular disease is a leading cause of death world wide (alternating with cancer for the top two spots). Congestive heart failure, hypertension, angina, cardiomyopathy, etc., all have their root cause in mitochondrial dysfunction. Not only is there a cellular energy loss, but also leakage of purines, which are the building blocks of ATP out of the cell (see details in the brain section below). The purines get metabolized to uric acid, so high uric acid as in gout reflects dysfunctional mitochondria.

In ischemic heart disease, there is poor blood flow to the heart muscle and poor oxygen delivery thereby causing angina. It takes several weeks to months for the heart to build up enough ATP by natural means to offset the deficit. Most patients will need to take targeted nutritional therapy and supplementation (i.e., D-ribose) to restore the energy balance.

All muscle contraction, whether voluntary skeletal muscle or involuntary smooth muscle, starts with calcium ions entering the myosin and is dependent on ATP. Relaxation begins with the removal of calcium and stimulation of an enzyme that deactivates myosin, and this process needs more energy than contraction. An illustration is the state of rigor mortis after death where muscles remain contracted without ATP. Magnesium is also necessary for muscle relaxation, without which the smooth muscle of blood vessels can't relax and hypertension is the result.

The same process occurs in heart contractions. Without adequate energy and magnesium the heart muscle can't relax properly and fill up with blood in the ventricles (diastolic dysfunction) and eventually become thickened (hypertrophy) and stiff, causing high blood pressure and less blood pumped out of the heart (low ejection fraction). Blood that backs up results in congestive heart failure. To prevent this scenario, abundant ATP must be ensured. The heart rhythm also requires energy for proper ionic balance, without which it becomes irregular (arrhythmia). All these functions are dependent on the mitochondria to make enough energy in the form of ATP.

BRAIN AND NERVOUS SYSTEM

The brain and nervous system also have a high demand for energy from mitochondria and have the lowest threshold for displaying symptoms (brain fog, poor memory, and cognition, etc.). In fact, the brain is 2% of body weight but consumes 20% of the total energy the body needs. The brain is estimated to have 100 billion neurons and several times more of glial cells that support them. Each neuron forms 10,000 connections to other neurons and 1,000 trillion synaptic connections, all forming a giant tangled network. It consumes 14% of the body's blood flow and 20% of oxygen, yet has a very small energy reserve of only about a minute. Therefore nerve cells are particularly vulnerable to low blood flow (ischemia) and low oxygen (hypoxia). When there is a blood clot or hemorrhage, the oxygen supply quickly runs out and the cells shift to anaerobic metabolism for a short time before suffering irreversible damage. The central area dies quickly, while the surrounding area is "stunned" and may be reversible depending on the mitochondria. These areas of reduced blood flow continue to generate free radicals and do further damage occurring days later, becoming a vicious cycle. In this situation, two ADP molecules are combined to form one ATP and one AMP. AMP can't be used by the cell and is eliminated, thus reducing the overall energy pool of the cell. The mitochondria go into a low-use state like hibernation.

Restoring blood flow is certainly the goal in therapy. But when blood flow and oxygen is restored, there is a greater injury to the mitochondria, called reperfusion injury. When oxygen returns, the mitochondria start to wake up but now there's a deficiency of the building blocks of ATP because they were thrown out of the cell as AMP. The result is a high rate of free radical production, which further damages the cells close to death and irreversible damage results. The delayed cell death probably happens by apoptosis. Delaying this process is critical to preserving brain function and nurturing our mitochondria may be the key.

NEURODEGENERATIVE DISEASES

In 1999 D.S. Cassarino concluded that functional alterations in the mitochondria can lead to pathological changes in neurons.[19] Neurodegeneration occurs based on a vicious cycle of mtDNA mutation, bioenergetic decline, and free radical damage. Abnormal mitochondrial function cause neuronal death and the onset of Alzheimer's, Parkinson's, and Huntington's disease. The brain is particularly vulnerable to free radical damage because of the high-fat content and a lack of antioxidative defense. The result is a gradual accumulation of oxidative damage to the lipid-rich membranes. Again, mitochondrial health is critical to prevent a decline in our mental state.

Excitotoxicity from overstimulation of nerve cells develops when the energy level of neurons decline. CoQ10 as a supplement can protect against this by raising energy levels in neurons. Glutamate as in MSG (monosodium glutamate) is an excitatory neurotransmitter and in neurodegeneration, the brain becomes oversensitive to glutamate. The mitochondria are constantly under command to produce more energy than they need, and over time burns them out from excess free radicals.

The presence of mitochondria at synapses improves the stability and strength of the nerve signals. In their absence, the signals they sent fluctuated greatly. Blocking ATP production also reduced the strength of the signals and have been implicated in major neurodegenerative diseases.

The amyloid plaques in Alzheimer's generate free radicals, damage mtDNA and alter protein folding to form neurofibrillary tangles. However, it is now believed the plaques are a defense against oxidative stress and pathogens that enter the brain and are a result of Alzheimer's, not a cause. Berger's research concluded that Alzheimer's is a metabolic disorder and we need a greater focus on mitochondria in the prevention and treatment of the disease. Cellular energy production is a better indicator of disease severity than plaques.

Another potent free radical called peroxynitrite formed from nitric oxide oxidizes lipids in the membranes of nerve cells. Its highly toxic metabolite hydroxynonenal (HNE) is found in excess in multiples regions of Alzheimer's patients. CoQ10 and vitamin E can protect cell membranes from this damage.

Overeating by consuming 2100–6000 calories per day may double the risk of mild cognitive impairment (MCI) in adults over age seventy compared to those consuming less than 1500.

Recent research in animal models of Parkinson's disease suggests that CoQ10 can protect brain cells from neurotoxicity. This draws attention to the importance of mitochondrial dysfunction and cellular energy in this condition. It plays a large role in the progression of the disease. Cell death is targeted to the neurons in the substantia nigra that produce dopamine neurotransmitter. Their death depletes dopamine stores and leads to muscle rigidity and tremors.

This part of the brain has the greatest number of mutations in mtDNA and several other deficiencies. There is diminished Complex I activity and increase in hydroxyl free radicals after administering L-dopa, which is the current conventional therapy, suggesting this may not be the answer. It is well known that L-dopa eventually loses its effect and the symptoms return with greater severity.

CoQ10 has proven neuroprotective properties that have helped neurodegenerative diseases. Administration of CoQ10 in rats showed its level rose by 10%–40% in the cortex to that of younger rats. CoQ10 also attenuated chemically induced neurotoxicity.

Depression is experienced up to 20% of the population. There is evidence that mitochondrial dysfunction and free radicals may play a role in mood disorders. In individuals with dysfunction, a stress-induced depletion of the brain's energy supply could render the individual vulnerable to depression.

Attention deficit hyperactivity disorder (ADHD) and autism spectrum disorder (ASD) are two other rapidly growing conditions in this country. Several studies have linked them with elevated oxidative stress and free radical damage from environmental pollutants, illness, or genetics.[20] Treating mitochondrial dysfunction might be beneficial. Cell death can also result from over-excitation from glutamate with excessive free radical damage and apoptosis.

CHRONIC FATIGUE SYNDROME AND FIBROMYALGIA

These are distinct and separate conditions with similarity and overlap in symptoms, so it makes sense to discuss them together. Fatigue, cognitive dysfunction, headaches, and sleep disturbances are common to both. Pain with pressure on the pressure points distinguishes fibromyalgia. They all have mitochondrial dysfunction and undersupply of energy as their root cause. They make a small amount of ATP by glycolysis (anaerobic metabolism), which can quickly generate some energy but are far less efficient than aerobic metabolism. This switch results in lactic acid buildup with muscle pain and chronic fatigue. Other brain and cardiovascular symptoms are also due to a mitochondrial problem.

MEDICATION-INDUCED MITOCHONDRIAL DISEASE

Medications can damage mitochondria both directly and indirectly. They can directly inhibit mtDNA transcription of ETC complexes and components or enzymes of glycolysis and beta-oxidation. Indirectly, medications cause mitochondrial damage by free radicals and decrease the number of endogenous antioxidants like glutathione. Barbiturates were the first medications found to inhibit Complex I. Other drugs can sequester coenzyme A (aspirin); inhibit the synthesis of CoQ10 (statins); deplete antioxidant defenses (acetaminophen); inhibit beta-oxidation enzymes (tetracyclines, anti-inflammatories); or inhibit oxidative phosphorylation (amiodarone). Some substances impair mtDNA transcription or replication. In severe cases, impaired energy production from acetaminophen could contribute to liver failure, coma, and death. Fortunately, the antidote is a common supplement called N-acetyl-cysteine (NAC), which is a precursor of glutathione. Many psychotropic medications also damage mitochondrial function. These are the antidepressants, antipsychotics, dementia, seizure, and mood stabilizers.

PRIMARY MITOCHONDRIAL DISEASE

When mitochondrial disease exists from birth, it is a primary disease. In mild cases, people adapt to the energy level they have, such as avoiding sports. Some have developmental delay or regression, seizures, muscle weakness, poor muscle tone, poor balance, cramps, low endurance, chronic fatigue, stomach problems, temperature and sweating problems, breathing and eye problems, loss of vision, droopy eyelids, deafness, tremors. People with mitochondrial diseases are usually affected by multiple symptoms at a young age.

Unfortunately, there is no cure, and treatments can't guarantee symptom relief or improvement in the quality of life. CoQ10 improves brain bioenergetics and significantly in muscle. All the supplements mentioned in Chapter Six can be helpful as a cocktail. Regular exercise and activity provide immense benefits as a way to build more mitochondria and can improve the quality of life.

AGE-RELATED HEARING LOSS

This condition known as presbycusis affects one-third of all people sixty-five and older. It's related to circulatory disorders that affect the brain and the auditory system such as heart disease, arteriosclerosis, diabetes, and sedentary lifestyle. New research shows that hearing loss is linked to cognitive decline. Animal studies show that the cumulative effect of free radicals could induce damage to mtDNA and eventual apoptosis of the cochlear cells of the ear. Exposure to loud noise can induce excessive generation of free radicals in the cochlea and can cause several genes to mutate, including those related to antioxidant defense. It's possible to slow and even reverse hearing loss using nutritional and lifestyle choices. Michael Seidman in his book *Save Your Hearing Now* revealed that hearing loss is linked to free radical damage and will the mitochondria start to multiply as the embryo grows. If she is female, her own oocytes will multiply tremendously to seven million. Then there is a purging of defective ones so that by birth she is down to two million. By puberty, she is down to three hundred thousand oocytes: survival of the fittest.

After the best reproductive age, a woman's CoQ10 declines, and less and less energy is made to the point where she is no longer fertile. In cases where there might be suboptimal energy but above the threshold for miscarriage, there are more birth defects like trisomy 21 (Down's syndrome) because there is insufficient energy to separate the chromosomes during cell division. Based on animal studies, it is recommended that women with age-related infertility supplement with CoQ10.

EYE-RELATED DISEASES

Mitochondrial aging is associated with the development of age-related eye diseases such as macular degeneration, cataract, glaucoma, diabetic retinopathy, and others. Macular degeneration is one of the most common eye diseases in the elderly and a leading cause of blindness. Free radical damage from UV and blue light with increased mtDNA and nDNA mutations and concurrent decrease in DNA repair contribute to this condition.

The retina (rods and cones) requires more energy per cell than any other tissue, so the number of mitochondria is also among the highest in the body. With age, the high-energy mitochondrial dysfunction. He showed a calorie-restricted diet can reduce free radicals and lead to a decreased progression of hearing loss. Another study showed acetyl-L-carnitine or alpha lipoic acid can contribute to an improvement in hearing.

AGING SKIN AND WRINKLES

The skin is the largest organ of the body and serves multiple functions: protects against external environment and pathogens, provides insulation, temperature regulation by sweating, detoxification, and synthesis of vitamin D. Research shows that impaired mitochondrial energy production plays an important role in the aging process. Fibroblast cells that produce collagen and elastin demonstrate dramatic mitochondrial dysfunction in aging adults. They are less able to carry out their functions and contribute to the wrinkling, sagging, and other aging signs. One source of free radical damage is from the ultraviolet radiation of the sun.

INFERTILITY

Mitochondrial DNA from the father is not passed on to the offspring, only maternal. The reason why mitochondria are so important in fertility is that each oocyte contains one hundred thousand mitochondria to serve the energy needs of the developing embryo. This is a huge number given the fact they remain dormant for most of their existence. In contrast, sperm cells only have a few hundred mitochondria but they are vital to their ability to fertilize the ovum.

To be motile, sperm cells need to have a very high metabolism, which results in free radical damage and mutations in their mtDNA. By eliminating this potential source of defective DNA, the oocyte prevents such mutations from being passed on. Soon after fertilization, any sperm mitochondria that enter the oocyte are engulfed by phagosomes resulting in autophagy. If autophagy is impaired, paternal mitochondria remain into the first stages of embryonic development.

Remember that building the complexes of the ETC require both mtDNA (encode 13 proteins) and nDNA (encode more than 800 proteins). But it's the mtDNA that's in charge because it codes for the critical subunits of the complexes. Once they are in place, it attracts the other subunits encoded by nDNA, and if they're a good fit, everything gets built properly. If they're not a good fit, energy production is compromised and the mitochondria or the cell may die. For this reason, ensuring only one set of mtDNA survives in the fertilized egg is very important.

Oocytes from women of advanced age show accumulations of mtDNA mutations. If they can't support the energy needs of the developing embryo, these eggs will be terminated resulting in a miscarriage.

While the embryo is rapidly dividing, the mitochondria do not. The original one hundred thousand get divided up so by two weeks; each cell has about two hundred mitochondria. Defective ones will be eliminated and that cell may die; if many are defective, the pregnancy is terminated. Only after all the defective mitochondria and cells have been eliminated demand and environmental assault produce significant free radical damage. This results in a 30% drop in the number of light receptive cells by age seventy, especially in dim light, making night driving difficult.

Glaucoma is the second leading cause of blindness. Half of the people with glaucoma remain undiagnosed. Here the free radicals damage the eye's drainage system and fluid builds up until the optic nerve is damaged by the pressure.

CANCERS

The orderly chain of events in apoptosis requires ATP. If the supply fails to meet the cell's demand, it cannot commit apoptosis. Deficient ATP production is due to mutations in either the mtDNA or nDNA or defective proteins involved in the apoptosis cascade. Mitochondrial function is in absolute control of apoptosis and prevention of cancers.

The mitochondrial involvement in cancer formation was discovered by Otto Warburg in 1930. Warburg discovered that when cancer occurs there's an increase in anaerobic glycolysis (fermentation) and gluconeogenesis (glucose made from non-carbohydrate sources) and decrease in the Krebs cycle and oxidative phosphorylation and fatty acid oxidation (burn fat).

Cancer cells have 220 times more mutated mtDNA than mutated nDNA. This is easily detectable in urine, blood, and saliva from patients with various cancers using rapid sequencing protocols. More than one thousand different proteins are found in mitochondria that can be measured. There is now an established mitochondrial protein database that will lead to the identification of markers for the detection of cancers.

The mtDNA mutations can be the target of anticancer agents. Several compounds have shown some degree of efficacy in killing cancer cells. Using light therapy, these compounds are concentrated into the mitochondria of cancer cells and converted to a more toxic compound without affecting normal cells. Other drugs are wrapped in a phospholipid membrane (liposome) that target mitochondria. The goal is to deliver drugs specific to the mitochondria whether to destroy dysfunctional ones or to replenish them with healthy copies of the mtDNA.

AGING

If mitochondrial dysfunction is at the heart of all the age-related diseases, then treating the dysfunction should be able to cure aging. The trouble is finding the mechanisms related to all the degenerative diseases, which are complex and numerous. There may be mutations in the protein subunits of the ETC complexes (either mtDNA or nDNA), defective autophagy, defective division or fusion, transcription, protein transport channels, protein assembly, permeability pores, apoptosis enzymes, enzymes of Krebs cycle or fatty acid oxidation, other organelles with which it communicates, etc. Obviously, we're still a ways away from finding the cure, but we're making progress with new technology. We should be able to extend the lifespan to 160 years in the near future and at that time new scientific discoveries and technologies will extend the number even further. We have to keep in mind the goal is to extend the healthy years and not just old age, which would be a huge burden on society. There are of course many ethical and practical questions we have to answer, but it's intriguing to know exactly how long humans are capable of living.

CHAPTER SUMMARY

1. There are more than 200 known mtDNA mutations that give rise to many common chronic diseases. Some exist at birth and are known as primary mitochondrial disease.
2. The initial symptoms are non-specific with fatigue, sleep disturbance, decreased endurance, mood swings, muscle, and joint pain. Later on, there is severe fatigue, brain fog, anxiety, depression, cardiac and respiratory problems.
3. Some of the more common conditions involving mitochondrial dysfunction are diabetes, cardiovascular disease, neurodegenerative diseases, cancer, aging, chronic fatigue syndrome and fibromyalgia, infertility, and loss of stem cells.
4. Age-related degenerative diseases like hearing and vision loss and skin wrinkling are also mitochondrial diseases.

CHAPTER EIGHT

ACTION PLAN SUMMARY

With so many options to improve the health of one's mitochondria, what is the best approach here? No single therapy is ideal, and it seems the best outcomes are from a combination of them along with exercise, which is non-negotiable. The best way is to try what seems feasible for you and do them consistently so they become a habit. Start by removing the toxins and chemicals that damage or block mitochondria from working. Then you can add in supportive supplements while you dial in the proper diet and healthy lifestyle habits. Keep adding items in each category until you have a well-rounded plan for total recovery.

MY ACTION PLAN

For me, during my health journey through musculoskeletal fatigue, I relied heavily on body works and bioenergetics, which made me feel more comfortable. I did infrared sauna three times a week followed by a quick cold shower. I liked red light therapy for areas of pain and on the face and body at night, which helped with sleep. I drank twenty-four ounces of hydrogen water daily and did aerobic and strength training three to four times a week to maintain muscle mass. I also did stretch exercises for leg and hip stiffness and weakness throughout the day. I grounded on a mat daily and at the beach several times a month and on vacations. I exercised using a mini-trampoline daily in the open air and sunshine, which increased agility and coordination in the legs.

Diet-wise, I kept to a paleo diet with low carbohydrates, moderate protein (mainly seafood), and quality fat. I had done a ketogenic diet for a few months and gluten- and grain-free diet which helped me lose 15 pounds, mostly in the belly. Now I have grain a few meals a week, mainly rice. I continue to do intermittent fasting of sixteen to eighteen hours four to five times a week. I tried one course of the fasting-mimicking diet (FMD) just to overcome the fear of fasting. Unfortunately, it made my thyroid function low and I was feeling cold through winter.

For supplements, I kept to a regimen of multivitamins, fish oil, CoQ10 (ubiquinol), PQQ, nicotinamide riboside, L-carnitine, magnesium, and NAC for mitochondrial health and biogenesis. I also did a combination of antioxidants like turmeric (curcumin), vitamin C, D, mushroom powder, resveratrol, berberine, milk thistle, gingko, and alpha-lipoic acid.

For those who sit at a desk job, it's really critical to get up every half hour and do some basic stretches to straighten the back and bend back the head. Too many people are hunched forward with head down in front of a computer, which straightens the natural curves of the back. Do a few bends and squats and walk around a bit. I paid dearly for not heeding this advice. My legs became so stiff after getting up from the chair it became painful to walk. I highly recommend getting an adjustable varidesk for the computer so you can work standing once in a while. Some get a treadmill desk so they can walk or jog while on the phone or computer. Or simply work standing up and walk or jog in place and do knee bends. What seems very basic can really harm our health when our hip and leg muscles either get too stiff or too weak and your entire legs get out of balance and cause myofascial pain. The muscles go into anaerobic respiration and the lactic acid buildup causes more pain and severe fatigue. We have to strengthen our muscles to have more mitochondria.

YOUR ACTION PLAN (DIY)

Keep in mind that base hits win the ballgame, but you have to have a game plan and follow through with action. According to Dr. Klinghardt, a world-renowned naturopath, the reason mitochondrial dysfunction is so prevalent today is they are poisoned from environmental toxins. Heavy metals and other toxic metals like aluminum are direct mitochondria toxins. Many intracellular infections can infect the mitochondria like mycoplasma and Borrelia (Lyme disease). So the first priority is to get the poison out before the supplements or nutrients can get into the mitochondria. Even with exercise, it doesn't work with someone with severe chronic fatigue since the mitochondria are too poisoned that they can't repair the muscle afterward.

If you're currently suffering from a mitochondrial dysfunction with fatigue, I recommend you start with regular sauna (dry or infrared) that helps you detoxify your toxic load. If you have a chronic infection like Lyme disease, mold, or gut parasite, you need to concentrate on getting rid of it first. Once the poisons of the mitochondria are removed, we can then support their recovery with supplements mentioned in Chapter Four. When you have more energy, you can start to improve your diet with a ketogenic and an elimination diet to find your food sensitivities. Eat as organic as possible to avoid pesticides, which poison the mitochondria and the microbiome. Now add in various lifestyle changes mentioned in Chapter Five. Among these, the most important is the circadian rhythm and exercise. Start slow with daily movements like walking and stretching and build up to HIIT and resistance training once or twice a week with rest days in between. You have to strengthen the muscles because that's where you have a quarter of the mitochondria. Breathing exercises and meditation or other stress relievers are also very important to boost your energy production.

If you're currently not suffering from a mitochondrial disease and want to prevent or delay degenerative conditions related to aging or want to biohack your way to longevity, you have the freedom to do as much as you can handle from diet, supplements, and lifestyles. Avoid exposure to chemicals and toxins in the air and water and personal care products. Detoxify at all times with saunas, hydration, and colon and liver/bile cleanse. Eat a plant-based organic diet low in grains and high in healthy fats. You must make some form of fasting and calorie restriction a regular part of your diet as it is the only proven way to boost mitochondrial function and biogenesis.

Start at whatever level you are at and build a program of constant improvement. Write in a health journal what you are starting and how you feel from it. If you feel improvement, stick with it and if not, try something else. Within a few weeks or months, you will have a good idea what you want to make into your daily or weekly routine. You don't have to do them all; do what is reasonable and affordable. The main thing is to constantly learn about the mitochondria and investigate what's new to fight against their dysfunction.

For supplements, start with a base of glutathione or NAC, CoQ10 as well as ubiquinol, and magnesium along with a quality multivitamin. Add in fish oil and L-carnitine, polyphenols, and an adaptogenic herb or mushrooms. Maintaining gut health is always central to your program and may include prebiotics, probiotics, and gut herbs. In fact, I would make gut health a lifestyle factor as it is the starting point of all chronic diseases. We are fortunate that there are so many things we can do today to help our mitochondria, which is at the center of our health and vitality.

CONSULT A FUNCTIONAL MEDICINE PRACTITIONER

When should you consult a functional medicine practitioner concerning mitochondrial dysfunction? I would say if you have any of the top five symptoms: fatigue, stress/depression, can't lose weight, gut issues, and hormonal imbalance. These symptoms often have mitochondria problems as the root cause. They may be slow (hypometabolic state) or there are not enough healthy ones (decreased autophagy and mitogenesis) from the environmental insults. Mitochondrial dysfunction also drives fragility and loss of resilience to age-related diseases and accelerated aging.

Inability to lose weight is a very common complaint. Although there are many causes, the inability to burn fat by aerobic respiration is one factor. Hormonal imbalance, particularly adrenal and thyroid hormones, is another. High toxic load is frequent and often not recognized. These have mitochondrial dysfunction as the root cause.

Hidden gut infection from bacteria, yeasts (Candida), and parasites often with no or vague abdominal discomfort is another frequent finding. Again, the mitochondria are compromised by infection and inflammation. You may be in the early subclinical stage of an autoimmune disease. Your practitioner can help you find these infections with functional testing.

As we have seen age-related degenerative diseases are all related to mitochondrial dysfunction. High toxic load can be assumed to exist until proven otherwise. Heavy metals and chemicals like plastics (bottled water, food wrappings, etc.)

build up in the body from poor liver detoxification, which ultimately leads to poor energy production. The overworked mitochondria can't meet the demands of the 247 pounds of toxins each one of us is exposed to per day excluding foods, pesticides, and drugs.

Oxidative stress is another major driver of mitochondrial burnout (my organic acids test showed I have it). There is simply excessive production of free radicals coming off the ETC that damages mt and nuclear DNA and other components of the mitochondria. Our excessive calorie consumption from sugars and carbohydrates is another factor contributing to oxidative damage. The abundance of processed foods lacking in micronutrients further damage energy production since it requires so many B vitamins and minerals to function properly.

Your functional practitioner can help you design a protocol that incorporates elements of all three categories. He or she can do annual functional testing to follow your progress. If there are reversals in your health, he can find the root cause and address it in a timely manner before it develops into something serious. The supplements we prescribe are for practitioners only and are of much higher quality. We also have access to the latest products on the market such as peptide therapy like vasoactive intestinal peptide (VIP) and BCP 157, which act as neuromodulators and decrease brain inflammation.

If your goal is healthy longevity without chronic diseases, a functional medicine practitioner can help you design a program for this as well. I particularly enjoy designing a longevity program since it is a current goal for myself and I enjoy sharing it with my patients and now the world through this book. The key is in the health of the mitochondria. Let's all set a goal to live to 120 or more and be full of energy and vitality up to the end!

REFERENCES

1. *Guntry, Steven. The Longevity* Paradox. New York: HarperCollins (Harper Wave), *2019.*
2. *Know, Lee. Mitochondria and the Future of Medicine.* Hartford, VT: Chelsea Green Publishing, 2018.
3. Naviaux, Robert. "Metabolic Features of the Cell Danger Response." Mitochondrion 2014 May: 16:7-17.
4. Whitten, Ari. "The Energy Blueprint Building the Cellular Engine (Hormesis)", www.theenergyblueprint.com. Accessed Sept. 2018.
5. *Seyfried, Thomas. Cancer as a Metabolic Disease.* NewYork: John Wiley & Sons, 2012.
6. Linnane, AW et al. "Mitochondrial DNA Mutations as an Important Contributor to Aging and Degenerative Diseases". Lancet 1989 March 25;1:642-5.
7. *Pizzorno, Joseph. The Toxin Solution.* New York: HarperCollins (HarperOne), 2019.
8. Picard, Martin. "Psychological Stress and Mitochondria: A Systematic Review". *Psychosomatic Medicine* 2018 February-March: 80(2):141-153

9. Bennett, Suzanne. *Mighty Mito: Power Up Your Mitochondria for Boundless Energy, Lazer Sharp Mental Focus and a Powerful Vibrant Body.* Wellness for Life Press, 2016.

10. Jockers, David. "How To Follow A Ketogenic Diet." DrJockers.com Accessed July, 2019.

11. Bénard G et al. "Mitochondrial CB1 Receptor Regulate Neuronal Energy Metabolism". *Nature Neuroscience* 2012 March 4.

12. Asprey, Dave. *Headstrong.* New York: HarperCollins (Harper Wave), 2018

13. Jenson, Nadia et al. "The Glymphatic System A Beginner's Guide." *Neurochemical Research* 2015 Dec 40 (12).

14. Ohsowa, Ikuroh et al. "Hydrogen Acts as a Therapeutic Antioxidant by Selectively Reducing Cytotoxic Oxygen Radicals". *Nature Medicine* 2007 May.

15. Kalish, Dan, Cutshall, Suzanne, Bergstrom, Larry. "Evaluation of a functional medicine approach to treating fatigue, stress, and digestive issues in women." *Complementary Therapies in Clinical Practice* 23 2016, 75-81.

16. Kalish, Dan. *The Kalish Method: Healing the Body, Mapping the Mind.* 2012.

17. Lord, Richard. *Paths to Health: Organic Acids.* iBook 2018.

18. Nagpal, Ravinder et al. "Gut Microbiome and Aging" *Nutrition and Healthy Aging:* 2018; 4(4): 267-285.

19. Cassarino, DS, Bennett JP. "An Evaluation of the Role of Mitochondria in Neurodegenerative Dis-

eases". *Brain Research Brain Research Review.* 1999 Jan;29(1):1-25

20. Giulivi, et al. "Mitochondrial Dysfunction in Autism". *JAMA* 2010;304: 2389-2396.

GLOSSARY

Adenosine: a compound present in the energy molecules formed by combining adenine with D-ribose.

ADP: adenosine diphosphate, the precursor of ATP.

Aerobic metabolism: energy production in the cell by using oxygen in the inner mitochondria membrane.

Antioxidant: a compound that protects against oxidation (free radical formation) either directly or indirectly catalyzing the breakdown of oxidants.

Apoptosis: programmed cell death or suicide to remove damaged cells or parts of cells.

ATP: adenosine triphosphate, the cellular energy currency, formed from ADP and phosphate on the inner membrane of mitochondria. Splitting ATP releases energy to power cell functions.

Autophagy: the "self-eat" orderly destruction of cells or parts of cells.

Beta oxidation: metabolism of fat into energy.

Biogenesis: new formation of cells or organelles like mitochondria.

Chromosome: a long molecule of DNA, either circular as in mitochondria or straight as in the nucleus.

Circadian rhythm: a natural internal process that regulates sleep and wake cycle in a 24-hour period.

DNA: deoxyribonucleic acid, the double helix structure containing genes which encode the sequence of amino acids in a protein.

Electron transport chain (ETC): a series of protein complexes on the inner mitochondria membrane that transport electrons by redox reactions that react with oxygen to form water and ATP.

Free radical: a highly reactive molecule with an unpaired electron.

Glycolysis: a metabolic pathway to convert glucose to pyruvate anaerobically.

Heteroplasmy: a mixture of two or more different mitochondrial DNA.

Hypoxia: a state of oxygen deprivation in cells or tissues.

Ischemia: reduced blood flow to a tissue or organ resulting in hypoxia.

Krebs cycle: is a sequence of chemical reactions by which aerobic respiration takes place in the mitochondria that convert acetyl-CoA into carbon dioxide and water with release of ATP.

Metabolic rate: the rate of energy production measured by oxygen consumption.

Mitochondrial DNA (mtDNA): the chromosome found in mitochondria, circular and from maternal source.

Neuroplasticity: the brain's ability to change throughout life to adapt to a changing environment to compensate for injury or disease.

Organelle: tiny organs within cells dedicated to a specific function, like mitochondria.

Proton gradient: a difference in proton concentration between one side of a membrane and the other by a proton pump.

Redox reaction: a reaction between two molecules where one is oxidized (lose an electron) while the other is reduced (gains an electron).

Uncoupling protein: a channel in the membrane that allows protons to flow back through the membrane, dissipating the proton gradient as heat.

ABOUT THE AUTHOR

Michael Chang M.D., CFMP, is a board-certified physician in Pathology and Laboratory Medicine and a certified functional medicine practitioner since 2012. He has a private practice Healed and Whole Clinic in Sunnyvale, California (Silicon Valley) since 2017, specializing in gut and mitochondrial health/anti-aging. He welcomes online consultations. His interest in mitochondrial health started during his mentorship with Dr. Dan Kalish, who emphasizes this area through his use of an organic acids test. During that time, he went through a health crisis with severe leg stiffness and fatigue. By doing the same testing and treatment plan for himself as for his patients, he was able to quickly recover after finding the root cause. Dr. Chang's goal is to empower his patients to be proactive in recovering their health and maintain it for the prevention of chronic diseases and prolonging longevity.

Dr. Chang is married to his wife Cynthia of thirty-six years. He enjoys traveling, classical music, and the arts.

ACKNOWLEDGMENTS

I would like to acknowledge all my mentors who have taught me functional medicine: Drs. Ronald Grisanti, Peter Osborne, Sachin Patel, and Dan Kalish. I want to thank my teachers and coach at Self Publishing School who gave me the idea to write a book and make it a reality. My editor Barry Lyons and Matt Stone for cover design and formatting. I wish to thank my patients for bringing functional medicine to life. Most of all to my wife Cynthia for her infinite support and understanding to make a dream into reality.

Thank You For Reading My Book!

I would appreciate receiving some feedback from my readers so that I can correct or add additional material for future editions of this book. Please leave me an honest review on Amazon as well as ideas for improvement that you may have.

Thanks so much!

Michael Chang

CPSIA information can be obtained
at www.ICGtesting.com
Printed in the USA
BVHW051407160721
612147BV00014B/1026